How to Talk with Family Caregivers About Cancer

How to Talk with Family Caregivers About Cancer

Ruth Cohn Bolletino

W. W. Norton & Company
New York • London

A Part of the How to Talk Series

Copyright © 2009 by Ruth Cohn Bolletino

For information about permission to reproduce
selections from this book, write to Permissions, W. W. Norton & Company, Inc.,
500 Fifth Avenue, New York, NY 10110

For information about special discounts for bulk purchases, please contact
W. W. Norton Special Sales at specialsales@wwnorton.com or 800-233-4830

Manufacturing by R. R. Donnelley Harrisonburg
Production manager: Leeann Graham

Library of Congress Cataloging-in-Publication Data
Bolletino, Ruth Cohn.
  How to talk with family caregivers about cancer / Ruth Cohn Bolletino.
— 1st ed.
      p. ; cm. — (How to talk series)
  Includes bibliographical references and index.
  ISBN 978-0-393-70576-8 (pbk.)
  1. Oncologists. 2. Caregivers—Counseling of. 3.
Cancer—Patients—Family relationships. 4. Communication in medicine.
5. Cancer—Psychological aspects. I. Title. II. Series: How to talk
series.
  [DNLM: 1. Caregivers—psychology. 2. Neoplasms—psychology. 3.
Family—psychology. 4. Psychotherapy—methods. QZ 200 B691h 2009]
  RC254.5.B65 2009
  362.196'994–dc22   2009014013

                ISBN: 978-0-393-70576-8 (pbk.)

W. W. Norton & Company, Inc., 500 Fifth Avenue, New York, N.Y. 10110
www.wwnorton.com
W. W. Norton & Company Ltd., Castle House, 75/76 Wells Street, London W1T 3QT

            1   2   3   4   5   6   7   8   9   0

To Larry LeShan,
who has taught me what it means to be a therapist
and all my clients
—people who have cancer and those who love them—
who teach me what it means to be a human being.
With gratitude.

RCB, 2009

Illness is the night-side of life, a more onerous citizenship.
Everyone who is born holds dual citizenship, in the
kingdom of the well and the kingdom of the sick.
Although we all prefer to use only the good passport,
sooner or later each of us is obliged, at least for a spell, to
identify ourselves as citizens of that other place.

Susan Sontag, *Illness as Metaphor* (1990, p. 3)

Contents

Acknowledgments

My special thanks to Larry LeShan, my long-time mentor, colleague, confidant, and friend, who sat with me over coffee and sandwiches as soon as a draft of each chapter was finished to read every word of it. His astute, informed comments and unfailing enthusiasm, guidance, and encouragement helped me always to move forward.

I also would like to acknowledge Sam Ellenport, who, despite knowing virtually nothing about psychotherapy or cancer (but a great deal about books and bookbinding), gamely and lovingly plowed through a version of almost every chapter and offered his unprofessional but valuable reactions and suggestions.

I want to express my thanks to my editors at W. W. Norton, particularly Andrea Costella, who invited me to write this book, which I surely would not have written otherwise.

My thanks, too, to all who formed my cheering squad, most notably Hannah Hendry, Sally Bergman, my niece Sandi Perlmutter, Kathy Gurland, and Jennifer Middleton, for reading parts of the work in progress and cheering me on.

To the caregivers and to the people they have loved and cared for who entrusted me with their stories and opened their emotional worlds to me, my deepest gratitude for making this book possible.

Introduction: Cancer Is a Family Illness

Our worlds are changed by the experience of illness and so are we indelibly marked by the ordeal, just as the heroes of Greek mythology cannot escape the underworld without paying a price or making a sacrifice. . . . No one returns exactly the same; there is a bitterness or compassion, strength or fragility, faith or despondency that was never there before.

Katt Duff, *The Alchemy of Illness* (1992, p. 18)

Most mental health practitioners have had little or no training or experience with clients dealing with cancer in the family. Yet at any time someone might turn to a therapist when their family member has been diagnosed—and they are suddenly required to become a caregiver.

A caregiver may be the spouse or partner of someone who is ill, or the adult child, parent, sister or brother, or close friend. Whatever the relationship, cancer is a family illness. For some families, the course of cancer is long and catastrophic. For others, it is comparatively brief or manageable. In any case, from the moment of diagnosis the life of everyone in the family, as well as the family structure, is changed, often forever. A cancer diagnosis has been likened to a bomb going off in the living room, leaving the house filled with debris and all its occupants damaged. How extensive the damage is or how long it lasts depends on how it is addressed psychologically as well as medically. It also depends on how cohesive the family is, how well family members can communicate, and how effectively they can adapt to crisis and change.

Cancer is emotionally infectious. The emotional responses of family caregivers are in many ways like those of the person who is ill. However, while family members and patients share many fears and feelings, the two are in different situations, with different experiences and reactions. While family members are usually caring and supportive, often they are overworked and overstressed. They are providing some degree of support, help, and care for someone suddenly dependent on them in new ways. At the same time they have to try to keep all the activities of daily life together, often taking over the responsibilities of the person who is ill. They might serve as companion, friend, counselor, nurse, aide, advocate, breadwinner, financial manager, secretary, care team manager, and surrogate decision maker. They handle household tasks, medical appointments, and child care, as well as rising expenses and falling incomes. With all this, generally they have little time or energy left for social contacts or activities that could help sustain them. In this situation, their relationship with the person who is ill can change dramatically. For everyone in the family the diagnosis brings new challenges, new frustrations, new roles, and new responsibilities. For everyone involved, the diagnosis is an enormous emotional assault. Often brokenhearted, confused, anxious, isolated, frustrated, resentful, guilt-ridden, and dispirited, family caregivers are at particular risk for numerous mental and physical problems, many of which have their roots in stress, exhaustion, and self-neglect.

This book is a guide for mental health professionals working with an individual family caregiver of an adult diagnosed with cancer: a spouse, significant other, sibling, adult child, or parent. The term *family caregiver* is intended here to refer not only to relatives, but also to anyone close to an adult cancer patient who provides nonprofessional care or support, such as a life partner or friend. The term *family* refers to the group of people closest to the patient, whether they are the family of origin or of choice. Although the therapist might meet at times with the patient as well as with the family member, this book does not deal with family therapy in which the therapist works with the whole family system. Rather, it is about helping practitioners ease their clients' emotional suffering, maintain their sanity, and find their own best ways to come to terms with their situation and with their own feelings and reactions. With this help, hopefully family members can deal with the illness and provide a healing environment for the patient, and the family can grow stronger, more cohesive, and more loving than before.

No two families are alike. They differ widely at least with respect to their structure and composition, their history, the nature of their relationships and interactions, their sources of strengths and tensions, their communication, values, perspectives, attitudes, and their reactions to the illness. Regardless of all their differences, the questions caregivers most often ask are, "How can I deal with this terrible situation? I'm terrified and overwhelmed" and "How can I help the person I love?"

The two parts of this book address these two major questions. Part I describes typical experiences of family members and offers a general approach for helping them cope with their situation. Part II suggests ways practitioners can help those clients support and care for the cancer patient in situations they are likely to encounter. The final chapter deals with ways that practitioners can prevent burnout when they work with people dealing with cancer, and with the rewards of this work. The book also includes appendices providing general background information for practitioners with little or no knowledge or experience in the fields of cancer and mind-body medicine.

Medical information is included only insofar as it bears on clients' common concerns. As a psychotherapist, I am rarely asked by family caregivers or cancer patients for medical information or advice. No mental health professional without an MD degree is qualified to provide it, so it would be unethical to offer any. Answers to questions about the medical aspects of cancer and treatment are available to patients and family members from their physicians and the Internet. However, while therapists cannot be expected to offer medical advice, in order to work with these clients they must be familiar with at least some basic facts about the nature of the illness and its treatments. Families dealing with cancer usually have certain fears and beliefs about cancer and its effects. Some are realistic, others completely unfounded. It is only with some knowledge about the medical issues involved that practitioners can begin to understand these clients' stories, respond to their beliefs and expectations, and deal with their emotional concerns. Basic information about cancer and treatments are provided in the appendixes.

Throughout I have tried to avoid or at least minimize the use of professional jargon in the hope that family members and cancer patients who pick up this book will find it clear and readily comprehensible. This style was chosen with professional readers in mind as well. Psychological terminology reflects an intellectualized, objectified view of clients and of the therapy process, a perspective not at all helpful in working with people facing a life crisis. Effective psychotherapy with these people needs to be, above all, a human relationship, driven not by concepts, theories, or techniques, but by these clients' existential concerns.

My clients' stories that appear throughout are accurate in all essential particulars, but have been altered in various ways to ensure their anonymity.

A Note About Pronouns and Perspective

At times throughout this book I will refer to the family member ("the client") or to the person with cancer ("the patient") as "he" and at other times as "she." For the most part, equal use will be made of both pronouns, although they will be chosen at random.

What is far more significant is that at times I use the pronoun "they" to refer to family caregivers or to the people with cancer they care for, and at other times the word "we." There is no real distinction between mental health professionals and the caregivers or cancer patients who are their clients. There is no "them" as opposed to "us." We are all in the human condition, just in different parts of it, and none of us can know what life will bring. Any practitioner might suddenly become a caregiver when a loved one is suddenly diagnosed with cancer (or perhaps you have already been one), just as any practitioner could become a cancer patient (or perhaps you have already been one). As professionals working with clients involved with cancer, it is very important that we are always aware of this, for it shapes our attitude toward our clients. It determines how we view and interact with them. If we choose to maintain "professional detachment" in our work with people dealing with a life-threatening illness, we might succeed in sparing ourselves some emotional pain, but we pay a high price: our work with them will be relatively ineffectual and, consequently, less gratifying. (One oncologist was well aware of this when he said to his patient, "The only difference between you and me is that I can still maintain the illusion of my invulnerability.")

I learned this very well a year after I began specializing in therapy with people with cancer and those closest to them when I myself was diagnosed with that illness. During my year of treatment (when, as some of my clients would put it, I was "slashed, poisoned, and nuked"), it became very clear to me that before that time, in my mind there was always a gap between them and me. We were different: they were sick and I was well. After my diagnosis, however, there was no gap. From my own experience with cancer and from my clients I learned a great deal about what it means to be human in times of great transformation. I came to different ways of seeing the individuals who were my clients, thinking about them, and working with them than what I was taught in the universities, the psychotherapy institute, and the workshops I attended. As a result, I became a much better therapist and my clients did far better as well.

People faced with cancer are forced to the awareness that death is real. As a result they take life very seriously. Priorities become very clear: In this situation we know what is important and what is not. In that heightened state we are in when we lose our delusion of invulnerability and face our mortality, we often find that we have a greater capacity for life and living, and more strength than we ever knew.

It is my hope that this book will guide practitioners in helping their clients recognize that capacity, and strengthen their sense of their inner being.

PART I

A GENERAL
PSYCHOTHERAPY APPROACH

CHAPTER 1

The Experiential World of the Family Caregiver: Where Psychotherapy Begins

The morning after an earthquake we learn about geology.
Ralph Waldo Emerson, *The Conduct of Life*

An earthquake is heard as a roar shaking the very foundations of the earth. There is an exploding, chaotic, colliding tumble of rocks from deep in the earth's bowels. Then there is stillness, as sudden and astonishing as what came before (Ascher, 1993). Hearing a physician say that someone we love has cancer is like that.

In the mornings and nights after a cancer diagnosis we find ourselves in a new emotional terrain.

Unless they have had the experience themselves, most practitioners know only in a theoretical way what it is like to have someone close to them diagnosed with a life-threatening illness. In almost all cases, the family's life is overturned, often suddenly, often dramatically. Like the person with cancer, family members are dealing with changes that can affect every facet of their lives. Watching someone they love go through a life-threatening illness can ignite nearly every feeling on their wide spectrum of emotions, certainly including those they would prefer not to feel. While they do not share the illness, they have their own kind of suffering. It is this that leads them to seek psychological help.

It is a simple matter to describe these family members (as well as the person who is ill) in terms of a standardized *Diagnostic and Statistical Manual* assessment (American Psychiatric Association, 1994). It is highly likely that almost anyone trying to cope with cancer can be diagnosed as having not one, but at least three kinds of mental disorder: an adjustment disorder, an anxiety disorder, and a depressive disorder. When it comes to trying to know and understand any individual, however, diagnostic labels tell us nothing. They serve only to categorize and stereotype these clients. If anxiety, depression, and an inability to adjust were not present before the diagnosis, they are certain to occur in reaction to it. If they are not present at all, something is very wrong with the client.

This chapter attempts to describe the typical experiential world in which people often find themselves when someone close to them has been diagnosed with cancer. Whether the patient is newly diagnosed, is found to have a recurrence, is in treatment, is not responding to treatment, or is not treatable, in many ways the emotional world is much the same. It is a world of turbulent, complex, and conflicting feelings, including fear, anxiety, resentment, anger, guilt, grief, helplessness, frustration, depression, and despair. Any of these feelings can arise again and again at any time, before and after these clients can come to terms with reality. In this situation, calmness is a way of coping, not a way of reacting. Underneath a calm surface, intense emotions often are boiling.

Like the patients themselves, family caregivers are often bewildered by their strong emotions, and think they should not be feeling as they do. They often believe that their intense reactions are abnormal or indicate weakness. Too often health practitioners mistake those reactions for psychological conditions that need to be worked with accordingly or medicated away. However, it is when someone in their situation does *not* react with intense feelings that there is reason for concern.

One purpose of this chapter is to normalize those reactions. If you are a practitioner who has never entered the world of cancer, it is one that you need to be very aware of, for it is the emotional terrain on which these clients live and on which your work with them takes place. Unless we have some sense of what our clients are experiencing, it is not possible to connect with them. Unless we comprehend their emotional world, we might think we are communicating with them in a caring, helpful way with our words and attitudes—but we are not.

For that reason, another purpose of this chapter is to convey far more than a conceptual or objective account of caregivers' experiences. It is to try to capture that experience, to bring readers into the client's world so that practitioners can see it as the client does. Each therapist will deal with clients' problems with her own modality and approach. No modality or approach can be effective, however, without an understanding of the worlds in which these clients live. Only by approaching the problems of cancer from the viewpoint of family members and of the person who is ill can professionals gain a deep understanding of what these clients face. Only with such a deep understanding of their distress can we help to lessen their suffering. The writer André Gide said that perhaps the most important thing is to be capable of emotions, but to experience only one's own is "a sorry limitation" (1892/1987).

There are no universal truths about the emotional effects of cancer. Each person's experience and reactions are intensely individual. Not everyone feels all the emotions described in this chapter. Further, the extent of family caregivers' distress depends on the patient's reactions, the site and severity of the cancer, the prognosis, the nature and effects of treatment, the duration of the illness, and the demands placed on them. For this reason, these descriptions are no more than generalities. A generality helps us to become aware of the ways that an individual is different from others, and ways in which the person is the same.

It is important to note that the reactions described are not sequential stages. Any of them can arise unpredictably into the foreground at any time.

This chapter describes the painful emotions that a life-threatening illness sets off, but these emotions are only part of the story. People dealing with cancer, both caregivers and patients, are entire human beings. Enthusiasm, expressions of love and caring, excitement, joy, humor, courage, and the determination to fight for life are as much a part of what happens in therapy sessions as what happens in the darkest hours of the night.

Cancer's Effects on Lifestyle

Cancer impacts nearly every aspect of the life of everyone in the family. It changes family members' functions, roles, dynamics, and relationships. The person who has been diagnosed becomes a patient, while others take over tasks and responsibilities that at least temporarily the patient cannot handle. Family members might have to shoulder new breadwinning burdens or rearrange their work schedules so that they can assist the patient with daily activities and provide physical care. They might have to schedule medical appointments and make travel arrangements. They might have to arrange for and oversee home health aides or household help. Cancer can cause enormous financial strain as it drains the family's financial resources when income is lost or medical expenses mount. Family members deal with greatly increased workloads and little time just for themselves. Cancer can deprive them of the very touchstones of their lives: activities they normally enjoy, care and attention they normally receive, and friendships that can sustain them, because now their time and attention must be focused on the patient instead. Besides overturning their daily life in the present, cancer can also change their expectations, hopes, and plans for the future. It can affect the patient's livelihood, employability, sexuality, fertility, and sexual potency, and can cause permanent physical changes. It can also lead to lasting changes in the family structure, lifestyle, and relationships.

David was diagnosed with chronic leukemic lymphoma when he was 35 years old, not long after he and Sheila had been married and their first child born. His health deteriorated quickly and he could no longer work. Sheila became the family's sole support. At David's parents' suggestion, the three of them moved in with David's mother and stepfather, who had both retired several years earlier. It was a difficult adjustment for everyone, made far more difficult because David soon became seriously ill. In their new home Sheila was away longer each day than before because she had to drive farther to get to and from her place of work. Ann, David's mother, took care of the baby while Sheila was at work, often getting up at night for the infant because Sheila was so tired and, at times, for David when he could not sleep. Jim, David's stepfather, drove David to all his doctor appointments and sometimes got up during the night when the baby cried so that his wife could sleep. During the days David spent as much time as he could with the baby, but most of the time he was in bed, "out of it," as he put it, in reaction to his aggressive chemotherapy. The four of them met with me because they wanted to discuss growing tensions within the family and attempt to resolve them. Jim described their lives by saying, "Everyone is constantly on a roller-coaster—way up when David feels better and way down when he feels sick again."

Whether family members provide care or engage others to do it, the demands on them and the resulting stress are much the same. The more severe the patient's illness and the longer it has lasted, the greater the stress.

Don's father, Ralph, 83, had advanced pancreatic cancer and was being cared for at his home by a team of health aides. Because Don's elderly mother was in a state of early Alzheimer's and his brother lived abroad, Don was the primary caregiver for both his parents. Every day after work, before going home to his wife and daughter, he traveled to their apartment to see them and oversee their care. Sometimes he had to miss part or all of a day at his office because he was needed to take care of some kind of situation that arose at his parents' home. He had contacted me requesting that I make a house call to talk with Ralph, who, he said, had recently expressed disinterest in living. When I arrived at the large apartment at the time of our appointment, Don greeted me at the door. He explained apologetically that he had to ask me to wait while he talked with a visiting nurse and his father's accountant before they had to leave. He led me through the large apartment. There were people, apparently aides and other helpers, in every room we passed. As he led me to a study where we could talk privately before I met with his father, we passed the door of a small room off the dining room where I caught a glimpse of Ralph lying in a hospital bed. A chair was on one side of the bed and a large oxygen tank was on the other side. Apart from that, the room contained only a table stacked with medical equipment. I waited in the study for nearly half an hour before Don finally was able to sit down with me. He slumped into a chair and rubbed his forehead.

"There's a lot going on around here," I commented. "How are you doing with all that you have to deal with?"

"There's so much going on all the time that I can never even think about that," he said, and went on to talk about his father.

Emotional Effects

After a cancer diagnosis, in many ways the emotional responses of family members are much like those of the person with cancer. At times they mirror the patient's emotions. But while family members and patients share many feelings, the two are in very different situations, having different experiences. Family members are trying to provide various kinds of care, help, and support and at the same time are forced to readjust their lives and maintain the necessary activities of daily living. The patients are trying to take care of themselves and also trying as best they can to keep their normal activities going, but they are concerned about their bodies and their health, about the possibility of dying, and about the meaning of their life.

Like the patients themselves, family caregivers go through a storm of emotions and mood swings that confuse, bewilder, and distress them. Most react with different feelings at different times during the course of the patient's illness, and even during the course of a day. They are taken over by different feelings that come and go for no immediate reason, some of them conflicting, for which they are unprepared.

Shock, Disbelief, and Denial

The first reaction of both patients and the families immediately after receiving the news of a cancer diagnosis is almost always shock coupled with pain. (Janet, whose husband was diagnosed with late-stage cancer, said, "*Shock* is too mild a word. It's like we have been thrown into a fire.") We feel like we are going through life in a haze, unable to absorb the terrible news. We are bewildered, unable to comprehend fully what is happening and what it means. We reject the diagnosis and feel mentally and emotionally paralyzed. This state of numb detachment, involving a refusal to believe the truth, is a necessary defensive reaction against overwhelming terror. When we have a physical wound, a protective covering (a scab) forms over it. As the body begins to heal the wound the protective covering drops away. Denial is a healthy reaction. It is a protective covering over terror until we are ready to deal with the full emotional impact of what has happened. (No one is so sick that they react calmly to a cancer diagnosis.)

Our initial terror stems from the fact that no matter how knowledgeable we are, our first reaction is to regard cancer as an inescapable death sentence. The diagnosis tells us that everything in our lives is closing down: our plans, our hopes, our way of life, and the life of someone whom we love and count on being with us. In that moment when we receive the news, everything we believe in and depend on is changed. Our denial might express itself in a variety of ways: "The test results are wrong," "This can't be happening now," "He can't be that sick; he's been so energetic and felt so good," "But she has always eaten healthy food, exercised, and meditated," or simply, "The doctor made a mistake."

Normally, as things settle down when treatment is begun, the shock wears off as we know better what is happening and find that the patient and we ourselves are dealing with it. We begin to grasp the fact that the patient might get well.

Denial can come and go long after the diagnosis. Family members might accept part, but not all, of the situation (partial denial), choosing to believe, for example, that the cancer isn't serious, that a recurrence isn't significant, or that the patient's illness won't involve major disruptions in the family's life.

Denial can also persist and become unhealthy. As a long-term way of coping, it doesn't work. The difference between healthy and unhealthy denial is that unhealthy denial manifests as an unwillingness to take appropriate action. For example, a family member might choose to believe that the illness is not serious, or that there is no other possibility than that everything will be all right. In the case of mutual denial, when the patient might be dying, the family will not talk about it or plan together to prepare for that possibility.

Beth, a young woman with colon cancer, said that after her surgery, her husband seemed to have no doubt that she was now perfectly well, and that she and their life together would continue exactly as before. When she tried to express her fears or her feeling that everything now seemed different, he just kept telling her,

"You're going to be fine." As a result, she felt isolated from him and terribly alone with her fears and concerns. To live with someone and not be able to talk about the most important thing in your world is indeed a terrifying and lonely experience.

Even after the truth of the initial diagnosis breaks through and is accepted, family members are often overwhelmed by unpredictable and bewildering emotions.

Fear

Fear and terror surface again and again. When, instead of our familiar world, we find ourselves in an ambiguous world unknown to us in which we cannot predict or control what will happen, we are afraid.

While patients are trying to deal with their fears, as caregivers we have our own. We are unprepared for what is happening, and we fear for the person we love and for ourselves. Every day we live with the possibility that the patient will die, and we cannot stop ourselves from imagining what that loss might be like. Our fears are added to the pain we feel when we see the patient hurting, weakened, and afraid, and we never quite succeed in avoiding our feeling of helplessness. We wonder: What is going to happen? How can I handle everything I have to handle, and what if I can not? What if I'm not strong enough? What will I do if this person I love dies?

The possibility of the patient's death makes us keenly aware of the fragility of life and of our own mortality, and that awareness intensifies our fear. Particularly if there has been any family history of cancer, we might become fearful about our own health.

Gale's husband, Ron, had mesothelioma, an incurable cancer caused by exposure to asbestos. (It was later discovered that his exposure had come from a slow leak in the ceiling of his office in the building where he worked.) The two of them had consulted medical specialists in several parts of the country, and Ron had undergone various kinds of conventional, experimental, and adjunctive treatments in an attempt to extend his life. They had two young children, ages 6 and 8. Once, when Ron was having surgery in another city, they sent the children to live with Gale's sister in a neighboring state for 3 weeks so that Gale could stay with him. Another time, when Ron was hospitalized for 10 days in the city where they lived, Gale was able to sleep in his hospital room. Every afternoon she traveled home to be with the children for a few hours after school. Every day she tried to arrange for another friend or relative to stay with them for the rest of the evening and overnight, and worried about them while she was away. (One day these arrangements failed. She called a neighbor, who came into the apartment to put the children to bed, and returned in the morning to give them breakfast, but they had to be alone overnight. Later that neighbor accused Gale of neglecting her children.)

When Ron was home, Gale shopped and prepared meals for the children and herself and made special meals for Ron. She took care of his medications. As he became increasingly incapacitated, she provided more and more care. For the first time, she also learned to handle all their finances. She also tried to keep up with the voluminous bills and insurance claims, answered the many phone calls they were receiving, scheduled visits from friends and colleagues, arranged medical appointments and trips to physicians' offices, supervised the woman who helped occasionally with housecleaning and errands, and tried to spend time as much time as she could with the children. Sometimes she had to get up at night to take care of Ron. Sometimes the children woke up and needed her. Every night when everyone else was asleep, even though she was exhausted, she stayed up, unable to sleep until long after midnight, playing solitaire on the computer to wind down and distract herself from the terrifying thoughts that threatened to overwhelm her. Her fear, grief, and fatigue all felt the same. Every week her exhaustion grew until she seemed to be operating on sheer nerve.

Anxiety

While fear usually relates to something specific, anxiety is amorphous: At times we feel that something we dread is going to happen, but we aren't sure what. As in Gale's case, our anxiety is fueled by thoughts that we have to do things we cannot possibly do, or that we have to deal with more than we can possibly handle. We feel anxious when we don't know what to do for the person who is so ill. We feel anxious whenever we wait to hear what the doctor will say. We feel a stream of anxiety along with fear when we think about the death of the person we love, or about our own death—and we can't help thinking about these things. We feel anxious because we don't know what the future will bring, and we fear the worst. Sometimes we know only that we feel apprehensive and don't know why.

Most caregivers are confronted with a variety of unending obligations, and with a great deal of stress, in the attempt to take care of the person who is ill and also keep everything at home or at work going. It often seems like we are forced to make immediate decisions constantly. We have far less support and help than we need, and very often the load feels intolerable. Meanwhile we are dealing with our fears of the unknown and with the patient's needs and frustrations. Constantly witnessing the patient's pain or discomfort creates anxiety and stress, and makes us feel afraid and helpless.

We feel ourselves to be at the mercy of outside forces over which we have no control, including the pressures of planning for treatment and care, scheduling and keeping medical appointments, and traveling back and forth between home and hospital. We try to accept the need to comply with other people's schedules and are often kept waiting. We wait for doctors to call, and we wait in offices and hospitals for them to see us. We wait for test results and expect the worst. We wait for a treatment to work, hopeful and fearful at the same time. We might be putting in long hours of nursing care and longer hours of paperwork. We try to keep up with the unending piles of insurance claims and try not to worry about all the days lost from work and the unending outflow of dollars, all too aware that we don't know when it will stop. Not knowing what will happen causes helpless feelings that intensify our anxiety.

Helplessness

Anxiety is sometimes related to helplessness, powerlessness, and a feeling of inadequacy. No matter what or how much we try to do to help, we feel that we have no control over the painful and seemingly erratic events that are occurring. We cannot fix the person we love, and so we feel powerless against the disease and against all the changes in our lives. Each morning we feel helpless because of the uncertainty we face that day. We always feel helpless at not knowing what the future, even the next day, will bring.

For many of us, helplessness is unacceptable—and therefore unbearable. We might try to keep our helpless feelings at bay by trying to fix or rescue or baby the patient, usually out of our need to do something and not be powerless. There are times we might even take responsibility for the ill person's moods and try to fix them—for example, by trying to cheer him up or by trying to talk her out of sadness or despair. Fixing might take the form of rescuing the family member who is ill by taking over responsibilities that should belong to him. With the intention of helping him concentrate on getting well, we might take over many aspects of his life, including making personal decisions for him.

We might find ourselves infantilizing the patient. Because he sees us as trying to take away more of his independence, he might get angry at us and refuse our help. We, in turn, might become resentful and tired of playing the role of parent, and we might turn on the person we love. In some relationships, just the opposite happens. Instead of getting angry, the patient might become overly dependent on us, expecting too much and making too many demands, so that cancer takes over our lives even more.

Some of us try to use denial to avoid our feelings of helplessness. The spouse who is unresponsive to the fears expressed by the cancer patient may be trying to avoid his own feelings of inadequacy that he cannot make the patient well. A spouse might try to avoid feelings of failure, for example, by blaming the patient or by withdrawing from her, by drinking too much, or by spending long hours away at work.

Despair

Our feelings of helplessness leave us devitalized and dispirited. Even while we continue to do all that we know to do to meet and even try to change the situation, at times we despair.

Grief

Another natural response is grief. We feel grief at the diagnosis, and at the pain, discomfort, fears, and frustrations the person we love is experiencing. We feel grief every time a treatment doesn't work, and grief that this person no longer can maintain the same functions and activities, so that our lives are no longer the same. We feel grief at all that we have lost. We have lost the healthy person we knew, the life we had, and our dreams of the future. We feel grief at all that we fear we will lose and at the recurring thought that we might lose that person forever. We feel grief at the loss of our sense of self, knowing that we can no longer be the person that the patient made it possible for us to be. Cancer shatters many of our beliefs about what our lives are supposed to be like, and we feel grief at that loss, too.

Isolation

We feel separate from all the people who are not dealing with cancer. Friends and relatives often say insensitive things that hurt us. Even if we try to talk with them about how things are for us, it is clear that they have no idea of what we are going through and what we feel. Our isolation increases when others avoid us because they no longer know how to be with us.

Anger

More often than we wish, we feel anger and rage: at fate, at the universe, at God, at the diagnosis, at the prognosis, at the medical professionals, at the unwanted and unending demands placed on us, at someone's unthinking words or actions, and, at times, at the person who is ill. We come to resent our helplessness that comes from trying to help a loved one overcome cancer. Our losses can make us angry, and we have lost much: the life we had, the relationship we had, the person we knew who is now ill, the pleasures we knew, and the time and freedom we had.

Linda, whose husband, Jake, was diagnosed with lung cancer, said she feels anger at all the people she sees on the street because they all seem well while Jake is ill and suffering. ("Why him?")

We are angry because we feel that life is not just, for we did nothing to deserve this. At the same time we cannot accept the idea that terrible things happen randomly. We need to look for causes, so we assign blame. We blame others, ourselves, even the patient. Our targeted anger often defends us by diverting us from our fears.

Sometimes our anger serves to defend us against sadness. How natural and easy it seems to feel anger—at anything, at anyone—because it is easier to have an external cause than to face our deep underlying sorrow.

Sometimes our anger is a defense against our dread at the possibility of losing someone who cares for us in many ways. We might think that we would not know how to survive without the person and feel angry that he is letting us down when we depend on him.

We feel resentment and bitterness at the diagnosis, at the uncertainty of the outcome, at the overwhelming demands placed on us, at the loss of our freedom to come and go and do what we want, at all that has been taken from our regular life, and at all the unwanted changes cancer has brought.

We feel anger at doctors—for not giving us straight information, or for giving us information we don't want to hear, for taking away our hopes, for not returning our calls, and for their apparent insensitivity to our situation and our feelings.

At times we feel angry at the person who is ill for getting sick, turning our life upside down. We feel angry at the patient because we feel so alone. We might blame her for bringing crisis and tragedy into our life. We might well resent her dependence on us, particularly if she has been strong and capable in the past. Perhaps we feel that the person has regressed to a state of greater helplessness than the illness warrants and could be doing more to help us with all we have to handle. At times we are angry because we have to do all kinds of things we never wanted to do. Perhaps we resent what we perceive as the person's lack of appreciation for all we are doing. With all this, at times we find ourselves overreacting to small annoyances and lashing out at anyone just to release our anger.

We recognize that at the same time the person with cancer is also irrationally angry at us, and that this anger can be set off by trivial things. Sometimes he is angry even at the encouragement we give him because he experiences it as nagging. We, in turn, bitterly resent his anger at us because we are working so hard and suffering so greatly because of him.

And then there are moments we don't speak of, when we wish it was all over. And these moments make us feel terribly ashamed and guilty.

Guilt

It is so natural to feel a great deal of guilt about our thoughts and feelings. We feel guilty because we are healthy and strong, while the person we love is ill, suffering, sometimes in pain, and might even die.

Frank talked about how guilty he felt when he didn't want to go to the hospital to visit his wife, Margaret, one afternoon. He felt guilty when he tried to take a day off from the whole business of cancer, or even when he just wished he could run away from it all. Sometimes, he said, when the situation and his feelings were too much for him, he just had to withdraw from her, and this increased his guilt.

Often as caregivers we feel guilty about being angry and resentful, or about what we didn't do, or what we did and regret. ("Why did I let myself get angry at her when she is so sick?" "Why didn't I insist that he take a vacation instead of working so hard?" "Why didn't I see this coming?" "Why didn't I make sure that he ate better or rested more?' "Why didn't I put aside more money so she wouldn't have had to worry?") Sometimes we feel guilty because we resent all that lies ahead that we know we must do. ("How can I resent this, when I am well?")

We might believe that if we provide good enough care, the person will get well and that the course of the illness depends on us.

When Bob was diagnosed with pancreatic cancer, his wife, Jenny, took care of everything—their home, their finances, the medical arrangements—and supported him emotionally in every possible way. She stayed with him every hour of every day, taking walks with him when he felt strong enough and watching television with him or reading to him in the evenings. She felt strongly that she wanted to give back for all the love he had given her for the last 20 years. When she arranged for an aide to stay with him for a few hours while she tended to errands, Bob complained that he didn't need anyone to be with him while she was gone. Despite his protests, she didn't want him to be by himself, so she stayed at home, rushing to the store only when he napped. She took no time for herself to be alone or to do anything she enjoyed.

Thus if the person is failing, we see that as being our fault. We might feel guilt at our inability to cure the person we love. We might feel guilt because however much we are doing or how tired we are, we feel that we aren't doing enough.

Matt and Lisa, both in their 50s, had been together for 12 years. From time to time they talked about getting married or living together, but neither felt the need to do so. Lisa was involved with her teaching at a high school and with church activities. Matt worked for a large corporation in a job that required him to work long hours and travel almost every week.

From the time Lisa was diagnosed with late-stage breast cancer, Matt made every effort to spend as much time with her as he could. As her illness progressed, he took more and more time off from work to be with her in the hospital, to help her at her home, or to research treatment options. When his manager complained that he was neglecting his clients, he explained the reason for his absences and said he intended to continue taking time off from work. Lisa's condition became critical. Her sister, who had not seen her for years, flew into the city. She said that the situation was clearly hopeless, arranged for Lisa's transfer to a hospice, and left. Because Matt was not a relative and did not have power of attorney, he had no legal voice in the matter. During the last days of Lisa's life, he rarely left her bedside. He called in friends from her church choir who prayed and sang to her. ("It was heartbreakingly beautiful," he said.) When she died, Matt handled all the arrangements and costs for her funeral and burial. Several days after the funeral, he returned to his office. His manager informed him that despite his excellent work record with the company, he might be fired because he had neglected his job.

Matt felt that he had failed Lisa. "She was always hopeful. Even when one treatment after another didn't work, even when there were no more treatment options, she believed she could beat the cancer. I wanted everything to be her decision, but it didn't work out that way. If I had just done something more or done something sooner, if I had been more aggressive with the doctors, maybe that would have made a difference. It weighs on me. I feel I let her down."

Perhaps our guilt is greatest when we find ourselves hoping that it will all be over soon. Those moments make us feel even worse, because we feel there is something terribly wrong with us. ("How could I have wished even for a moment that she would die and get it over with?")

In short, we might find many reasons to blame ourselves: for not doing enough, for not loving enough, or, perhaps most of all, for not being able to take away the patient's illness and suffering.

Self-blame is a recurrent theme, and possibly the most common theme upon which we spin endless variations. It is a major way we wound ourselves, and those wounds can be damaging. We forget that we react as we do simply because we are part of the human race.

Emotional Numbness

From time to time, we feel drained and feel nothing. Separated from all our feelings, we function on automatic. Those times are welcome respites from the storm.

Ambivalence

Like the patients we are concerned about, caregivers often have ambivalent feelings and attitudes. Sometimes we feel one way, and other times the opposite. We are likely to respond with different and apparently conflicting feelings at various times during the course of the illness, or even during the course of a day or an hour. Sometimes we voice or act out one side, while the person who is ill expresses the other.

One form of ambivalence is optimism versus hopelessness. One spouse might feel hopeful when the other feels despair. One might be positive, optimistic, and determined, while the other is negative, pessimistic, and depressed. It is natural to vacillate between both and important that neither person denies their negative feelings. (Once, working with a man with cancer and his wife, I asked them, "Which is better—to be hopeful and hopeless together, or separately?" The couple began to laugh. The question forced them to look at their behavior objectively.)

There are many other kinds of ambivalence. One is taking action versus remaining passive. At times the person with cancer might do everything possible to try to feel better and get well; at other times he might do little or nothing to try to help himself. Another ambivalence is being nice versus being angry. At times a family member may want to comfort and support the patient in every possible way; at other times she might be irritated and resentful.

Conclusion

It is very important for practitioners to understand that most family members, like the person who is ill, generally are psychologically healthy and normal. They come to therapy for help because they are hurting. The emotions discussed in this chapter are reactions to the situation they are in. They are natural human responses to the traumatic situation that these people are trying to handle and often go hand in hand with resilience and strength. Sometimes family members seek help because they are afraid that their emotions will interfere with their functioning, rendering them unable to deal with the illness or with what they have to do in their lives. In any case, these caregivers can be helped.

If their emotions are not expressed, it is not because they are not felt, but almost invariably because they are hidden. Sometimes people hide them from others, primarily from the person who is ill, as well as others closest to them and their health care practitioners. They fear that others would not be able to understand their feelings, would not know how to deal with them, or would be burdened by them. Very often they feel that their reactions are signs of weakness or pathology, and that they should not be having them. In that case, the resulting guilt increases their ordeal of suffering.

Unless we practitioners can ask, "How do you feel about what is happening to you?" and then stay still and wide open to hearing the answers, we are isolating the patient further.

To enter willingly into the emotional world of people dealing with a life-threatening illness is a painful and difficult task. It is very natural for us to want to accept and even encourage our clients' cheerful façades. To enter that world over and over again often seems more than we can bear. Yet, if we are truly to be with our clients, ease their loneliness and pain, and help them, we must at least summon up the courage to try.

The first step is to try to feel and understand their experience.

CHAPTER 2

Putting Traditional Approaches Aside

To be sure, theory is useful. But without warmth of heart and without love it bruises the very ones it claims to save.

André Gide, *Journals*

The goal of therapy with family members is not to cure psychological problems. They are suffering because their lives have been overturned. For this reason, many of the traditional ideas and methods of psychotherapy do not apply.

Psychotherapy began with Freud, who was a doctor—a neurologist—before becoming a psychiatrist. Following the medical model, he regarded his work as scientific research. He considered his ideas as hypotheses to be explored, and his clinical work as investigation. A number of his ideas, however, have been absorbed into many forms of present-day therapy, often treated as dogmatic presuppositions, or axioms, assumed without question to be true, necessary, and helpful for anyone.

Many of his concepts and related methods are not appropriate for therapy with people dealing with the crisis of cancer. They are at least irrelevant, often ineffectual, and can even be psychologically damaging. To help these clients it is necessary to put aside a number of the traditional Freudian concepts in which many psychotherapists have been trained.

This chapter discusses some of these concepts underlying many different kinds of therapy today, and the reasons they are unhelpful for people dealing with a life-threatening illness. Not all forms of psychotherapy are based on these premises, nor do they shape the perspective and clinical approach of all psychotherapists. However, some of them are assumed to be true and necessary sometimes without being questioned or even recognized. It is always hard to see one's own presuppositions and even harder to see that in some situations they might be limited in scope or even inapplicable. By bringing our assumptions into the light, however, we can examine them. When we do, sometimes we can get a very different perspective. In the children's classic *The House on Pooh Corner*, A. A. Milne's character Winnie-the-Pooh discovered this:

> Pooh began to feel a little more comfortable, because when you are a Bear of Very Little Brain, and you Think of Things, you find sometimes that a Thing which seemed very Thingish inside you is quite different when it gets out into the open and has other people looking at it.

This chapter attempts to make some traditional and prevalent assumptions explicit, bringing them out into the open in the hope that practitioners will consider their appropriateness for each individual client.

Presupposition 1: Clients in psychotherapy can be viewed, classified, and treated in terms of mental disorders.

Freud was the first thinker whose concept of human nature was derived not only from theory but also from his clinical practice. From work with his patients, he developed his concept of human nature and a clinical approach that he and others believed fit all human beings. All his patients demonstrated neurotic behavior, and his work was designed for personality problems—for dysfunction and pathology. According to Freud, exactly the same underground forces operating in people who think and behave abnormally are at work in everyone: the difference between pathology and normality is only one of degree. In other words, people who display neurotic or even psychotic behavior are driven by the same forces as all human beings, but in them these forces are magnified and their effects are more pronounced. Thus from people who were mentally ill, he drew conclusions about people who were mentally healthy (Glaser, 1975).

Freud looked at his patients from the perspective of a physician whose focus is on pathology. The physician, looking for physical problems and their causes, asks three basic questions. The first is, "What is wrong with this patient; what are the symptoms?" For example, the physician's patient might be complaining of fever or pain. The second question is, "What are the hidden causes?" The physician would look for such causes as an infection or a broken bone. The third question is, "What can be done to fix the person?" For the physician, fixing might entail removing the cause or helping the person compensate for it (LeShan, 1994). The physician would try to eradicate the infection with medication or set the broken bone.

This same basic approach for medical problems is the one most prevalent in psychotherapy today. Therapists look at clients in terms of what is wrong with them, how they got that way (what the hidden causes are), and how they can be fixed. The assumption is that something specific is psychologically wrong with people that causes them to react and behave as they do—that is, that they suffer from mental disorders analogous to physical disorders that can be identified and treated. Patients have the same belief. They often come to therapy presenting their problems or symptoms with the expectation of engaging in a search with the therapist for the hidden causes of what is wrong, usually by exploring their past.

The problem with this approach for people involved with cancer is that as a general rule, there is no more psychologically "wrong" with them than with the rest of us. Like cancer patients themselves, family members are a cross-section of the general population. Usually they do not have mental disorders. Their psychological symptoms are natural, even predictable, reactions to the crisis of a catastrophic illness in their lives.

As discussed earlier, they often experience and exhibit anxiety, grief, and depression. Although these reactions arise after and as the result of cancer in their family, they can accurately be labeled with a *DSM* diagnosis (American Psychiatric Association, 1994). They are likely to have an anxiety disorder, perhaps even a depressive disorder. Chances are that they can also be diagnosed with an adjustment disorder. (Most mentally healthy people have problems adjusting to the fact that someone they love has an illness threatening their life.) While these diagnoses serve for insurance purposes, they are only vacuous labels when it comes to working with the client.

The attempt to understand healthy human beings in terms of pathology is inadequate as an explanation of human life.

Presupposition 2: Diagnosing the patient will lead to the cure.

When physicians go about trying to diagnose patients' problems, they are looking for a physical cause. Usually a medical diagnosis can be made, for which there are standard methods of cure. For example, when a patient's symptoms are diagnosed as having been caused by an infection, the physician prescribes an antibiotic and the infection is eradicated. When abdominal pain is diagnosed as appendicitis, surgery can remove the diseased appendix and in a short time the patient returns to the state of health experienced before the appendix became inflamed.

This is not the case with psychological problems and diagnoses. *DSM* diagnoses are very different from medical ones. While it might take some time and testing for a doctor to arrive at a diagnosis, most physical problems can be accurately described and diagnosed. Either a patient has an infection, a ruptured appendix, or a malignancy, or not. Psychological diagnoses are not like that: most psychological problems cannot be described adequately in terms of the *DSM*.

Further, identifying a family caregiver as anxious and depressed implies nothing about what that individual needs in therapy. It provides no information about the individual's total personality of which the anxiety or depression is a symptom. Neither does applying a diagnostic label help the therapist to better understand the client.

Often, in the beginning of therapy, many clients appear to fit neatly into a diagnostic category. However, this is because the therapist does not yet know them. It is unusual, even rare, to encounter an individual who clearly falls into a *DSM* category. Most people have a mixture of "symptoms." In the case of family caregivers, they come to therapy because their entire lives have been overturned. There is no classification for mental reactions to a devastated life.

While *DSM* diagnoses are necessary for insurers, in this case they are not helpful for clients or therapists. They can even hinder therapy. The therapist's first task is to get to know the individual who is their client. If they already have a diagnosis in mind, chances are that they will focus on apparent symptoms of that diagnosis and ignore or fail to see much else—possibly everything else—about their client, and thereby fail to see the person at all.

Presupposition 3: The roots of psychological disturbances are in childhood.
Presupposition 4: For that reason, therapy needs to focus on the past.

Traditionally, much of psychotherapy has been devoted to helping clients gain insights into the past causes of their feelings and behavior. The assumption has been that psychological problems in the present are the results of traumatic, psychologically destructive experiences or conflicts in early childhood. It is believed that by excavating and understanding those early experiences that formed the roots of the psychological problems, the client will be cured of symptoms, much like someone given antibiotics for an infection or an exorcism for a possession. This focus on the past is believed to help all patients whatever their issues, whether they are presumed to have a mental disorder or not.

However, family members seeking therapy are distressed in response to situations in the immediate present. Usually the roots of their emotional problems are not in the past. They need to be seen and responded to as they are now. Their concerns are about how to deal with what is happening in the present and about what they will do in the future. That is precisely where the focus needs to stay.

There are exceptions. Some family members bring past experiences to bear on the current situation of a family member's illness and see it from that perspective. Notable are those with a history of victimization or other trauma and those who experienced a recent or unresolved loss of someone close to them. These people are likely to see and react to the present situation in terms of the past. In this case exploration of the past is helpful insofar as it can separate past experiences from what is happening now. It also gives the therapist a broader understanding of the person. However, even with family members who have experienced loss or trauma, focusing on their past, particularly with the intent that they gain insight into what is wrong with them, is not helpful.

Presupposition 5: The goal of therapy is to bring about a cure. This can happen when clients can identify and understand the past causes of their psychological symptoms.

The traditional assumption is that through various processes (such as free association, interpretation, and dream work) clients can discover past causes of their present problems and that when these causes are recognized, the symptoms disappear.

In physical medicine, a cure is brought about by applying standardized procedures that stop the presenting symptoms. However, this is not what a cure means in therapy with family caregivers or other clients.

People dealing with cancer in the family are very aware of the causes of their distress. They are suffering because someone they love is ill and could die, and everything in their own lives is changed. Insight into painful childhood experiences will not cure the problem.

Even insight into why they feel as they do provide only part of a solution, for it does not help them change the fact that they still feel that way. Neither can it change the present situation to which they are responding.

The goal of therapy with these and, for that matter, other clients is not a cure, in the medical sense of the word.

Presupposition 6: Human beings are ruled by unconscious forces that determine their thoughts, choices, and behavior. Presupposition 7: Coming to understand our unconscious conflicts and discovering their historical causes can ameliorate and even cure the symptoms.

From his work with people who were psychologically ill, Freud drew conclusions about people who were psychologically healthy. Apparently it was for this reason that he and his followers regarded all human beings as ruled and driven by inner forces beyond their awareness and control. According to this theory, there is one psychological mechanism in particular that leads to neurotic disorders: repression. When we experience an instinctual desire (usually sexual) that conflicts with social or moral norms, we can put such an impulse out of consciousness—that is, repress it. However, the repressed impulse does not disappear. It is expressed through neurotic symptoms. Thus we find ourselves behaving in ways we do not understand and cannot control. For this reason, the theory goes, it is highly important for people in therapy to become aware of their unconscious motivation. This can happen through transference to the therapist, as well as by dream interpretation, free association, and slips of the tongue. Traditionally, unconscious conflicts often are regarded as more important to consider in therapy than conscious and present-day problems.

There has been much controversy about this idea of a dynamic "shadow mind" that, unknown to the person, rules or at least strongly influences thoughts, emotions, and behavior. Although everyone has thoughts and emotions that are out of awareness to some degree or other, it is not at all apparent that understanding their own unconscious motivations leads anyone to be able to live in a more fulfilling way. However, even if the idea of a dynamic unconscious is accepted, it is not useful in therapy with family members in crisis. Spending time in therapy with these clients looking for unconscious conflicts and delving into their historical causes is not what is needed. They have more than enough conscious conflicts to handle.

Presupposition 8: Therapists should reveal as little about themselves as possible.

This supposition is based on an early idea that clients project onto their therapists the same attitudes and reactions they had to their parents or others close to them in their childhood when their problems originated. The theory is that by becoming aware of the transference in therapy, they can come to understand their past, and through this understanding become able to undo long-standing patterns of destructive attitudes and behavior. Thus, it is believed, to best facilitate the transference, therapists are never to show their individuality. Rather, they are to behave like blank screens or ink blots onto which clients can project. By being anonymous, they can be seen as being anyone. Although the theory behind this is long out of fashion, some residue of the model of the opaque, mysterious authority figure remains.

It is a strange idea that clients dealing with cancer, who often feel isolated and in desperate need of connection, can be helped by a detached, unknown, anonymous figure. It is hard to see how maintaining an emotionally distant, objective attitude can be at all conducive to helping these clients. A therapist who is emotionally detached appears to the client to be uncaring—and then the client is alone.

Presupposition 9: Without a neutral, scientifically objective perspective, therapists are unable to understand and work with their clients.

Many therapists assume that they need to be emotionally detached, to distance themselves from their clients' emotions, in order to work effectively. Perhaps they have been trained to think that their proper role is to be a blank screen. Perhaps they fear that if they are their real selves, they might act out or harm their patients, or that the patients will see that they are immature or inexperienced and lose faith in them. These concerns are pointless. If a therapist is indeed harmful, hostile, or immature, patients are likely to know it. If they do leave in those situations, it is not a bad thing (Jourard, 1971).

Some therapists might not want to relinquish their appearance of authority and omniscience, on the grounds that this is what makes their clients feel secure. From Freud therapists have inherited the concept of "resistance," clients' unwillingness to be themselves. Instead it might be useful to think of resistance in the therapist, for in their attempt to maintain objectivity, therapists surely resist their own naturalness and spontaneity (Jourard, 1971).

Whatever the concern or rationale behind therapists' detachment, there are major problems with it. When they wear a mask of impersonality, hiding from their client without being genuinely themselves, they are modeling the same behavior that is symptomatic of many psychological problems. They are also reinforcing the isolation for which the client sought help.

Surely it is the therapist's task in any kind of therapy to draw the client's real individuality and personality—the client's essence, so to speak—into the therapeutic relationship. However, this cannot happen without letting the therapist's own real personality become involved as well. What this means is that scientific detachment or objectivity can at times be the antithesis of therapy (Ungersma, 1961).

Another problem is that without feeling and reacting in response to our clients—in other words, without empathy—we cannot begin to comprehend them. If we try to view human beings objectively, their entire essentially human dimension is lost to us.

This consideration cannot be expressed more clearly than it was by the psychiatrist R. D. Laing. He wrote that to look at a person objectively, as a scientist would, "is to cancel the live presence of the other person. To look at the other as an object is not only to change the person to a thing but, by the same token, to cut off, while one is so looking, any personal relationship between oneself and the other" (Laing, 1982, p. 17).

Presupposition 10: Psychotherapy primarily involves techniques.

The supposition that therapy consists of prescribed techniques is related directly to the previous one. If therapists remain detached in an attempt to maintain objectivity, they are not reacting naturally, openly, and spontaneously to whatever is happening in the moment. In that situation, their only tools, the only ways they have to respond, are standardized, prescribed techniques.

Therapists in training are taught ritualized actions that have been found to work, and practice them until they have mastered their use, much like a music student practicing scales. But this is not an accurate analogy. The music student is working toward the strength and dexterity needed to play music, not to perform scales. The therapist is simply rehearsing a script.

While psychotherapy surely has technical aspects, there is no evidence and no reason to believe that the use of techniques helps clients (or therapists) to grow. Rather, clients are more likely to feel manipulated. Furthermore, techniques are standard procedures, intended to be used with any clients. The problem is that the use of prescribed techniques ignores the individuality of each client. While the therapist who uses techniques might be behaving in a technically correct manner, one can only wonder how effective such generic therapy can be.

Techniques were devised to apply specific theoretical approaches. For example, the "empty chair" technique is an application of Gestalt theory; the technique of interpretation is an application of the psychoanalytic theory of repression and the unconscious; conditioning techniques reflect behaviorist theory; and the reflection technique is an application of Carl Rogers's approach. Every therapy approach is the outcome of a theory about the self and the human mind. The history and literature of psychology contains a plethora of such theories, which go in and out of fashion. Psychologists disagree about which one is correct—perhaps because none of them applies to everyone.

So if the therapist is not required to maintain a detached, objective stance and does not rely on techniques, what is it that guides the therapy process? The next chapter deals with this question.

CHAPTER 3
_____

Principles of Psychotherapy
With Family Members

The flow of therapy should be spontaneous, forever following
unanticipated river beds. It is grotesquely distorted by being
packaged into a formula . . . The therapist must strive to create
a new therapy for each patient.

Irving Yalom, *The Gift of Therapy* (2003, p. 34)

Family members who come for therapy might be the main source of
support for the person who is ill, while their own lives have been shattered. In response to this situation, their sense of independence, individuality, and control might well be eroded.

The goal of therapy with these clients is not to cure long-standing
psychological problems. It is to help them reorient their view of themselves and their relationships so that they are better able to recognize
their own sources of strength, adjust to the changes in their lives, and
solve their problems.

This kind of psychotherapy is guided by concepts or principles that
define an approach and shape the therapist's attitude. Concepts, as the
philosopher Ernst Cassirer has pointed out, are tools. We use them but
are not always aware that we do. In our work as psychotherapists, it is
very important to be conscious of the underlying concepts we use. If

we are not aware of our assumptions, we might use a sledgehammer when we should be using a tiny screwdriver—and then wonder why someone gets hurt. These guiding principles are the basis, the foundation of everything therapists do. They serve as axioms that define the way we think and the way we see and interact with clients who entrust themselves to our care. This chapter presents three fundamental principles or presuppositions of an effective approach for working with people dealing with the crisis of cancer. They are the essential axioms of this kind of psychotherapeutic process.

Presupposition 1: Each client is an individual—a total human being like no other.

Every person born into this world represents something new, something that never existed before, something original and unique.

Martin Buber, *Hasidism and Modern Man* (1990)

Every client needs to be viewed this way, and seen and responded to as a total person (LeShan, 1992). When we look at the person, we should be able to recognize that they broke the mold when they made her. It is as if, to paraphrase James Thurber, "Someone came into the room who closely resembled someone that no one had ever seen before." To be sure, in some ways all human beings are the same, but in very important ways we are all different from one another. As Dr. Eric Cassell put it, "Although we are flung into a torrent not of our choosing, once in it we determine our own ways of swimming through it—we individualize our route" (1994, p. 166).

A therapist's first session with a client is like starting the first page of a novel by Dostoyevsky or Tolstoy and then waiting to find out what happens. It takes a long time to get to know any human being. Slowly, very slowly, we come to get a sense of the personality and complexity of the person and of what his experience is like. This means that learning facts about a person's social or psychological history (the facts required to fill out a form) tells us nothing about who the person is, what he is experiencing, what matters to him, or who he might become. Without knowing these things, we cannot help. Without coming to know the person as an individual, we can only violate him. The psychiatrist Kurt Goldstein expressed this very clearly when he said, "Before I see a patient, I close my eyes and repeat three times, 'Now I must give up all my preconceptions'" (LeShan, 1996, p. 9).

Practitioners might find it convenient at times to assume that a client who has certain characteristics can be presumed to have certain others, but this is simply not the case. A story is told about another psychiatrist, Abraham Meyerson, who made this point to his students when he advised them: "As soon as you have decided on the basis of long experience and theory that all patients who have A also have B, and that this can be absolutely depended on, you can be completely certain that within three days a patient will come into your office with A and not the slightest sign of B. This will happen. The only question is, will you be too blind to see it?" (LeShan, 1996, p. 54).

It is so simple to view a person as a client or a case, or as an example of a set of symptoms or a diagnostic category, or as a depressed and frightened spouse, parent, or adult child. It is just as easy to see or think of the person who is ill as a cancer patient, a stage of an illness, a diseased body part, a survival statistic, or as someone who is terminal. Health practitioners of all kinds often look at patients this way, not only when they diagnose or treat them but also when they relate to them. We often see only what we are trained to see and ignore all the rest. It is much easier and less frightening to hide behind these abstractions than to open oneself to an encounter with a living human being.

Carl Jung was well aware of all this when he wrote,

Experience has taught me to keep away from therapeutic "methods" as much as from diagnoses. The enormous variation among individuals . . . has set before me the ideal of approaching each case with a minimum of prior assumptions. The ideal would naturally be to have no assumptions at all. But this is impossible. (1978, p. 81)

Studies have shown that when we look for something specific, our attention is volitional. We focus only on what we are looking for or expect to see and miss other things. It is so simple for any therapist to look at clients in terms of a diagnosis and to ignore the large number of ways in which they do not fit diagnostic criteria. All we have to do is to focus on what is wrong with the person and disregard or minimize what is right and unique. The problem is, if we do this, we are missing a lot. We are missing the whole person.

A useful rule of thumb is that the more closely a person appears to fit a *DSM* classification, the less we know about him. Lawrence LeShan teaches his supervisees another guideline which was provided to him by his training analyst, Joseph Michaels: when you see two patients whom you think need the same treatment, you're making a mistake about one of them. When you see three, you can be sure that you are treating them for your problem, not theirs.

Another way to ignore family members' individuality is to confuse their natural reactions to the illness with such psychiatric conditions as depression. Medical practitioners often fail to recognize that fear, grief, anxiety, and despair are natural responses to a catastrophic illness, and that pathology might lie in *not* having such reactions. Too often health professionals (including physicians), confronted with a patient's grief or depression, conclude that the person is chronically or clinically depressed and needs to be treated accordingly—usually with medication. Being depressed is not pathological when the person has something to be depressed about. Anyone facing a crisis like cancer who isn't depressed from time to time is the one who might well have a mental disorder.

Jane, whose college-age son Jason had cancer, knew how to deal with this. She told me that during an office visit with Jason's oncologist she started to cry. The oncologist looked alarmed and tried to stop her. She said, "Doctor, I'm just crying, not hemorrhaging."

Dave, a client of mine with a late-stage form of cancer, was more involved with life and living than almost anyone I have ever known. Even when he became very ill, he was more alive than most people ever are. (I have rarely seen anyone eat a slice of apple with more enjoyment than he did.) Because of the nature of his cancer, he and his wife, Margaret, feared that he would eventually face excruciating pain. His oncologist had treated him for several years and knew them both very well. When Dave began deteriorating rapidly and there was no longer any doubt that his condition was incurable, he tried to discuss with the oncologist his thoughts about the possibility of suicide. His doctor shut off the conversation abruptly, telling them that Dave was clinically depressed.

Anyone can be classified as a man or a woman of such-and-such an age, of such-and-such a weight and height, in such-and-such a profession. How does that work as a description of you as an individual? What does it miss? When we classify a client, that is precisely what we are missing: all the rest.

In short, everyone is far more than a set of psychological or life problems. Each person brings to therapy his own personality, his own values, his own way of viewing the world, and his own way of reacting to what life brings. Effective therapy rests on an awareness of the individuality of each person and a respect for her unique identity.

Particularly when we are dealing with a catastrophic illness that weakens the client's self-identity, each person needs to be seen and responded to as a unique, whole individual.

Presupposition 2: No psychological theory applies to everyone, and there are no techniques that are effective for all clients.

Learn your theories as well as you can, but put them aside when you touch the miracle of the living soul. No theories but your own creative individuality must decide.

Carl Jung, *Psychological Reflections* (1978, p. 84)

For effective therapy with people in crisis, there are no techniques. Because each client is unlike any other, there cannot be any effective preprogrammed methods, no one size that fits all. There are no standardized, routine procedures for any kind of real human contact. Contrary to many therapists' training, there is no one correct way to be with and talk with other human beings, and this is never more true than when they are under mortal stress.

Psychotherapy training and literature contain a profusion of technical approaches. They include, to name only a very few, interpretative techniques, conditioning techniques, reflective techniques, and Gestalt techniques. Students learn and rehearse them, and try to master them so that they can apply them almost mechanically. However, when therapy is regarded as a matter of applying techniques, the therapist's job is to be a technician, a mechanic, and the patient is seen as a broken machine to be manipulated and repaired (LeShan, 1982). At the right moment in therapy (which is always unpredictable), the right technique can do wonders and, as Jung pointed out, it is important that therapists learn their techniques well. However, psychotherapy is not a way of using techniques: it is a way of being with another person (Jourard, 1968).

It is the client that is of paramount importance, not a technique. We need a different language for every individual.

Just as no techniques fit every person or every therapy situation, no one psychological theory explains everyone. Since its beginnings, the field of psychology has been replete with theories about the self, most of them at odds with others. How do we know which is the most useful one for any individual client?

In short, there is no best kind of therapy, no best kind of approach for anyone. There is surely no best approach for someone dealing with cancer. Nearly all therapists have been taught that there is one best kind of therapy approach: the one taught by their school or their mentor. However, with different clients and with the same client at different times, different approaches can be helpful. The "right" approach depends on the individual and the moment.

Rather than techniques or theories, psychotherapy with people dealing with cancer is driven by these clients' immediate existential concerns. The therapist needs to be responsive to their vulnerability and to the urgency of their situation. It requires openness, flexibility, and authenticity. This means that the model of the therapist as a blank screen or a detached, objective observer simply does not work.

Presupposition 3: The therapist must be genuine and emotionally involved.

It is more by being than by doing that the meaningful and deeply felt communion between us and our patients will emerge. This demands as much honesty and freedom from us as it does from our patients, and as much trust on our part as we would someday hope to receive from them.

Robert Coles, "A Young Psychiatrist
Looks at His Profession" (2002)

When therapy is not based on techniques, what is left is the therapist himself, being himself, and engaged in a human relationship. This means being spontaneous, affected by clients' problems, and even at times willing to suffer with them. As Sidney Jourard once put it,

Effective therapists seem to follow this implicit hypothesis: if they are themselves in the presence of the patient, avoiding compulsions to silence, to reflection, to interpretation, to impersonal technique and kindred character disorders, but instead striving to know their patient, involving themselves in his situation, and then responding to his utterance with their spontaneous selves, this fosters growth. (1964, p. 62)

The intent of such therapists, he continued, is to use themselves in the service of their clients' well-being and growth, not to inflict anything on them. On the other hand, those therapists who confine themselves to thinking and only thinking beings are not likely to promote their clients' growth.

Being oneself in the presence of people dealing with cancer in their family is in some ways simpler than with other clients. With many other clients, the therapist often needs to go far beneath their habitual social or defensive masks. This takes time and work. The masks have become so ingrained that the persons behind them are hidden not only from the outside world, but also from themselves. Removing those masks to reveal the "real" self behind them becomes part of the psychotherapeutic work. However, when people confront such catastrophic events as cancer in the family, their facades usually drop away quickly. I see my clients struggle to express who they truly are in their shifting worlds. They haven't the time, energy, or interest for false fronts. Because their priorities and values are likely to have changed and become very clear to them, there is no point in trying to maintain a facade. The face they show to the therapist very early on is the real one. Their outer and inner selves have become much the same. Their feelings are very close to the surface, visible on their faces and expressed in their words. They are without pretense. As a result, they usually have razor-sharp antennae for other people's false words or actions. Therefore, the best and perhaps the only way for therapists to gain their trust and to reach them is by being authentic, too.

Therapists' responses and self-disclosure are bound only by ethics (at the very least, those of professional codes), by common sense, judgment, and the goals of the work. They might laugh, scowl, scold, joke, lecture, become annoyed, give advice, say what occurs to them in response to the client—in short, break many of the formal rules laid down in their training. Those formal rules can be discarded only when they are so familiar that they have become part of the therapist's being.

The only way we therapists can be aware of clients' feelings is to be aware of our own. At the same time, however, it is necessary that we discipline our feelings in the presence of the strong feelings of our clients. We must subordinate them so that we can see the clients clearly (Cassell, 1991). This is not a simple matter, and requires much training, supervision, and experience with a broad array of people. For therapists it is a personal goal well worth striving for.

With time, therapists usually can come to trust their own judgment and reactions more and more. They gain confidence that their spontaneous words will not harm the client, impede the therapy, or detract from their unwavering purpose of promoting the client's well-being and growth.

Self-disclosure is a matter of judgment. The criteria are always whether in some way it is supportive and strengthening to the client, and whether it furthers the relationship, the work, and its aims. The therapist's candor serves as a model. After all, we are asking clients to be as open as possible. This invitation rings hollow if we ourselves remain detached and defended. Just as candor serves as a model, so do boundaries. I do not hesitate to answer questions about my professional background, particularly about the kinds and duration of my personal therapy and supervision. While I will answer certain questions about myself—for example, where I was born, whether I am married, whether I have children, whether I am straight or gay, whether I have read certain books or liked certain films—some questions are simply out of bounds. To those questions, the response, "I would rather not answer that" will usually suffice.

There is a special caveat to self-disclosure with clients whose lives involve cancer. Almost inevitably, their stories and emotions arouse strong reactions in the therapist. (Therapists who do not get emotionally upset should not be doing this work.) Expressing most of these reactions is not in the clients' interests and could easily even be detrimental to the relationship and the work. In particular, if the therapist feels fear or horror in reaction to what the client relates about the cancer patient, pity (rather than compassion) for the client or the cancer patient, or any emotion in reaction to triggered memories of the therapist's own past, this is the time to become a silent, blank screen.

Work with people dealing with a life-threatening illness forces therapists to face their own vulnerability and mortality, and to confront their own past losses and grief. That is why psychologist Lawrence Le-

Shan described therapy with these clients as being "grown-up time" for therapists and strongly advised that they have more therapy or supervision, no matter how experienced they might be (1996, p. 37). (Dealing with reactions these clients evoke in their therapists is discussed in the Epilogue.)

The physician Eric Cassell expressed his conviction that doctors need to drop their professional armor with patients, surely including those who might be dying. In his now-classic book *The Nature of Suffering*, he wrote:

> One cannot avoid involvement with the patient and at the same time effectively deal with suffering. . . . To be concerned is to be involved. . . . Every physician has the same fear—becoming closer to suffering patients, many of whom will die, surely promise pain, sorrow and loss. Why would we not want to hold back, cover our feelings with a white coat, and hide behind incomprehensible technical language? Because, as understandable as self-protection may be, it renders useless the tools necessary for the care of the very sick and suffering. (1994, pp. 248–249)

Those "necessary tools" come from an emotional connection from which we can try to figure out what it feels like to be that person. With that connection, as Cassell put it, we can provide "a bridge over which the fragile person can return from the isolation of suffering, start to become whole again, and, through the relationship, reconnect with the world" (1994, p. 249).

The guiding principles discussed in this chapter can be summarized easily: Therapy that helps people deal with the crisis of cancer needs to involve two human beings in a human relationship. Unless we practitioners can say to these clients, "How do you feel about what is happening to you?" and then stay wide open to hearing the answer, we are further isolating the client.

The benefits to clients from their therapists' willingness to open themselves to the possibility of emotional distress are clear. But what do therapists gain by taking this risk? Seasoned practitioners learn from experience that the more open and unconcerned with self-protection they are, the greater the rewards. They find that being open does not damage them. Being concerned and engrossed makes the work both challenging and fulfilling. Deep rewards come from being in a real communion with our clients and, in so doing, learning more about what it means to be a human being.

During the last months of his life, writer and literary critic Anatole Broyard wrote about his experiences as a cancer patient. In one of his eloquent essays he said that practitioners need to see that their "silence and neutrality are *unnatural*" and advised that practitioners might have to give up some of their authority in exchange for their humanity (1992, p. 57).

When we do, we usually find that, just as he predicted, it is not at all a bad bargain.

CHAPTER 4

Toxic Myths

*Alice laughed. "There's no use trying," she said. "One can't be-
lieve impossible things."*

*"I daresay you haven't had much practice," said the Queen.
"When I was your age I always did it for half an hour a day.
Why, sometimes I've believed as many as six impossible things
before breakfast."*

Lewis Carroll, *Through the Looking Glass*

There is no way to know exactly how many impossible things people
can believe, but it is all too clear that too many people believe impossible things about having cancer for far longer than half an hour a day,
and not only before breakfast.

All human beings have beliefs about what happens to them. Most
such beliefs are unexamined assumptions or presuppositions that filter
experience. While many of these assumptions aid in survival, some can
be destructive. There are a number of widely held beliefs about cancer
with no basis in reality. They not only color and darken the experience
of patients and family members, but also define their attitudes and the
resultant behavior that can impact the patient's health.

Four such myths are particularly prevalent, high on the list of most popular destructive beliefs. Despite all that has been written in the field of mind-body medicine, I continue to hear them far too often from both family caregivers and cancer patients and, as a result, continue to spend an unfortunate amount of time trying to dispel them.

These beliefs are as harmful, as malignant, as the disease itself, with no basis in science or reality. At any time a client might express any of them explicitly or make a statement that presupposes its truth. From the first session the practitioner needs to be alert to hearing them. Whenever and however these beliefs are expressed, they are injurious to whoever holds and espouses them. Besides their psychological effects, they can affect the family's medical decisions and thus even the outcome of the illness.

This chapter discusses these four mythic beliefs in some detail. Any of them needs to be addressed soon after it comes to light: challenged, clarified, and corrected or reframed with more realistic and helpful concepts. Otherwise, the therapy is severely hampered (Bolletino, 2004).

Myth #1: People cause cancer.

The caregivers' version of this toxic notion is, "I could have done something to prevent this from happening." (The patients' version is, "I did something to cause my cancer.")

From a number of books on pop psychology, health, self-help, spirituality, or cancer survival, readers often come away with the idea that people cause cancer in themselves or others, that they could have prevented it, or that they are at fault for not conquering it. It is not unusual for caregivers to entertain the insidious idea that if they had acted differently in some way, the patient would not have gotten cancer, or would already have been cured. It is not unusual for cancer patients to believe that they are ill because of something they did or failed to do. Some family members believe that the illness was caused by some distressing event that they or the patient should have been able to control—even though in reality no one had control over it.

Some of the literature suggests that cancer occurs because of some kind of physical, emotional, or spiritual defect in the people who are ill. If their weaknesses can just be set right—for example, by means of forgiveness, raw food, body work, love of themselves or others, exercise, acceptance, wheat grass, laughter, relaxation, raw vegetables, prayer, meditation, or sweet thoughts—the illness will be cured. The assumption is that patients are responsible for their cancer, and that if they are not getting well, they are culpable for that, too. If they continue to hold negative thoughts, to feel unhappy, or to eat the wrong foods, they will also be responsible for dying. Caregivers sometimes apply this idea to themselves. They think they did something to cause the patient's cancer, and that if they can manage to act or feel differently and help in the right ways, the person will be cured. The inevitable result is that if the patient does not get better, they blame themselves.

Despite all evidence and arguments to the contrary in professional and popular mind-body literature, this belief—that somehow people can cause cancer in themselves or others—endures. One reason for its endurance is that it cannot be proven to be false. If the patient's cancer progresses or if a treatment doesn't work, this proves only that the person did not try hard enough, wasn't good enough, or didn't really want a cure to happen, not that their belief was wrong (Dossey, 1992).

Another likely reason that this idea persists is that we tend to look for simple causes for what happens to us. We need to make sense of our suffering. When catastrophic events occur (like earthquakes or cancer), we look for a reason. We seek explanations because if we see the universe as being rational and orderly, then we can believe that we have power over our lives. We want to deny that some things happen that we can neither understand nor control. Chaos and random tragedy are too frightening to contemplate. Assigning blame—in this case, to the patient or the family members themselves—is much easier and brings with it some sense of security that we have power over events that in reality are not in our control.

Magical thinking is involved when a family member says or implies that the patient's illness is his (the caregiver's) fault, or that he could have done something to prevent it. In response, I ask how he thinks he caused it. To this question I have heard all kinds of creative answers, including, "By trying harder to stop him from eating junk food," "By not insisting she leave that job she hated," "By agreeing to his going back to work after only a week off instead of taking a longer vacation, even without pay," and "By not going ahead and scheduling a doctor's appointment for him when he felt so tired." Patients' answers to the same question are at least as creative. I have heard such responses as, "By not having a positive enough attitude," "By not meditating (or doing visualizations or exercising) more (or better)," "By worrying (or feeling anxious, depressed, stressed, or angry)," "By not coming to therapy sooner," "By staying in a stressful relationship (or job)," or "By not eating more vegetables."

Because people who carry this belief hold themselves or someone else personally responsible, on top of the heavy burden of the illness they add guilt and shame. They think the illness appeared because of something they did or didn't do, once or habitually. With all of this they are not unlike people in ancient civilizations who believed that when their crops failed it was because they hadn't prayed enough to the gods. Whatever cause they assign, their guilt itself becomes a problem. If the cancer is not disappearing, they blame themselves for that, too, and see the illness as their personal failure. Cancer then becomes the punishment they deserve for something they did wrong. Some people see it as their punishment from God. It is sad and frustrating to try to convince people already dealing with more than they can handle that they are not at fault.

The professional psycho-oncology literature includes a variant of this belief in the form of theories of "the cancer personality." Advocates of these theories suggest that people who repress or discount their emotions, particularly anger or stress, are far more prone to getting cancer. So far, none of the studies of personality types and cancer have demonstrated any such causal connections, and in my own work with cancer patients I have seen no evidence that this idea is true.

The Reality: How to Respond

No one is talented or powerful enough to cause cancer.

We might be sufficiently skilled to give ourselves a virus, a cold, flu, or any other contagious disease and then spread it to someone else. We might trip someone and cause them to break their ankle. If we eat foods that are not nourishing but can be harmful instead, if we don't exercise enough, if we stand in front of an open window in the winter and then take a cold bath, if we live a life that doesn't fit who we are and that wears us down, or if we have no goals that are meaningful to us, we are indeed likely to be more prone to getting ill. Numerous studies have shown that chronic stress plays a significant role in many kinds of illness. In any of those situations, the immune system is weakened. As a result of a compromised immune system, we might develop pneumonia, ulcers, or high blood pressure. When our self-protective and self-healing abilities function at a low level, we also have an increased susceptibility to colds or other illnesses. Everyone surely has the ability to undermine or subvert their health in many ways, but there is a world of difference between neglecting our health and causing cancer.

Some contributing causes of cancer are known, but no disease, including cancer, has a single cause. Even when certain risks can be identified, they themselves do not invariably produce cancer (Matte, 2001). Tobacco, for example, is implicated in certain kinds of lung cancer. Alcohol has been linked to certain kinds of carcinomas, and skin cancer to overexposure to the sun. However, many people who smoke and drink heavily for most of their lives die of old age. Some people who spend half their lives in the sun do not get skin cancer. The sexually transmitted human papilloma virus (HPV) has been tied directly to cervical cancer, but some women with cervical cancer have been celibate nuns. Stress can contribute to lowered resistance to many kinds of illness, notably heart disease. It exerts an effect on the heart rate, hormones, and blood pressure. However, it is not at all apparent that stress is a direct cause of cancer. Besides, no one can avoid stress, and yet not everyone gets cancer.

"People become ill, not just because of germs, carcinogens, viruses, trauma, or stress, but because these assaults fall upon receptive hosts" (Jourard, 1964, p. 142). It has not been determined what causes any individual to have cancer. Apparently it results from some combination of genetic, environmental, and psychological factors. This view reflects the biopsychosocial view of illness: that illness, as well as health, results from the total individual and the individual's total environment.

Nothing can be done to change anyone's genetic heritage. We can control our environment, but only within limits—for example, by improving our diet or stopping smoking. Psychological factors alone, thoughts and feelings, do not cause cancer and cannot cure it. They are just one aspect of the total person. To be sure, feelings affect body chemistry (which affects the development or regression of tumors), just as body chemistry affects feelings, but we do not know how large a part the psychological factors play. Even if that part is only a very small one, psychological factors are the ones that can be changed. We can change them by changing the way we live. When we change the way we live and the things we do, we feel differently about ourselves. By changing our lifestyle and the way we feel about ourselves, we are changing the total environmental context in which the cancer grew—and thereby improving the likelihood of getting well (LeShan, 1994, p. 25).

Laura, in treatment for breast cancer, asked, "If I don't believe I caused my cancer, then how can I believe that I can do anything to cure it?" Now, there is a certain logic to this, but besides being a toxic idea, its logic is fallacious. Many things happen in life that we did not cause but can nevertheless change. Laura thought that if she was not responsible for getting cancer, she could have no control over its course. However, she was mistaken in this. There are better, less punishing ways than harboring such a belief to come to realize that there are many things patients and their families can do.

People who hold the destructive belief that cancer is God's punishment for something that they did or failed to do are seeking causal explanations for an unfathomable event. One wonders what kind of punitive God these people have in mind. Besides, terrible things happen in life that we can neither prevent nor control. Whether we like it or not, some events appear to be random, beyond our understanding or control. Since pain and suffering are such natural, even inevitable, parts of life, it is curious that these people think of cancer as a special punishment designed just for them.

We resist the idea that some things that happen to us are random events. We look for causes instead, even if it involves holding ourselves responsible, for we learned to think of the universe as a rational, orderly place. If events occur randomly, that means that our habitual view of the way the world works has to change. It also means that we have no control over what happens to us. However, the idea that cancer just happened, that it was a random event, is in fact an answer to the question why, an answer that can bring comfort. It means that no one is to blame. It means that cancer happened even though the patient and family members did everything right.

The prize-winning writer Audre Lorde, who died of breast cancer, wrote about this insidious belief in a book about her experiences after a mastectomy:

> The idea that the cancer patient should be made to feel guilty about having had cancer, as if in some way it were all her fault for not having been in the right psychological frame of mind at all times to prevent cancer, is a monstrous distortion of the idea that we can use our psychic strengths to help heal ourselves. This guilt trip which many cancer patients have been led into (you see, it is a shameful thing because you could have prevented it, if only you had been more . . .) is an extension of the blame-the-victim syndrome. It does nothing to encourage the mobilization of our psychic defenses against the very real forms of death that surround us. (1980, p. 74)

What is important is not what caused someone's cancer, but what can be done about it so that the person can get well. Although many things in our life happen that we cannot control, there are also many things we can change. Cancer is a disease of the whole person. Its course can be affected with an integrated approach that includes medical treatment combined with lifestyle and psychological changes. That is not just a theoretical possibility, but a conclusion from years of mind-body research and clinical observations that leave no doubt of this. There is a great deal that patients and their families can do to affect the course of the illness by means of the medical and adjunctive treatments they seek, and their attitudes, beliefs, actions, and expectations. Everyone has strong, highly developed self-healing forces operating to maintain or restore their health. These forces can be strengthened. There is much that patients can do to find ways to make their present experience have meaning and, as is discussed later, much that their family members can do to help.

Myth #2: The cancer patient needs to maintain serenity and to stay positive at all times.

Another popular destructive belief is that people with cancer will make themselves sicker if they allow themselves to have any so-called negative emotions, such as fear, anger, or grief. One problem with this is that it is not at all clear what they are supposed to do with such feelings. Apparently (to use the language in which this idea is usually couched) they are supposed to just "let them go," "detach," and then "get on with life." Precisely how anyone is supposed to get beyond these empty words to accomplish this, however, is not usually explained. Self-styled pop-spiritual gurus who advise us to think positively are notoriously unhelpful.

Many family caregivers hold this belief that people who are ill should remain tranquil, optimistic, cheerful, and upbeat, and that if they don't manage to do this—that is, if they allow themselves to harbor negative thoughts or to feel despair—they will not get well. This notion, too, arouses guilt and a feeling of failure in patients who find it difficult to maintain serenity in the face of an illness that threatens their life.

Besides the impossibility of remaining untroubled in the face of cancer and the resultant guilt at letting down their family if they do not succeed, there are other problems with this idea. First, it invalidates patients' natural reactions. To try to remain tranquil, it is necessary to suppress other, very different kinds of feelings. The result of the attempt is passivity. While patients try to remain calm and passive, another process is at work: their innate drive to act, to do something in response to a threat. So they find themselves in an emotional double bind. Either they say or do nothing and try to stay serene, or they act by expressing their true negative feelings in some way. When one option (remaining serene) is not possible, and the other (expressing real feelings) is unacceptable, they can only feel utter helplessness and despair (Dossey, 1992).

Also, since emotions are natural reactions to what is happening, the attempt to ignore or suppress them can be a way of avoiding reality. This is true of family members as well as the patient. When it comes to cancer, the failure to react and act can be harmful to themselves or others. Believing they should maintain a positive attitude, they are less likely to reach out for emotional, physical, or even medical help and support. Cancer in the family is a time for honesty, if only so that both patients and their family members can get all the help they need. Besides, when family members hide their natural feelings by maintaining a cheerful facade, they themselves pay a high psychological price and the patient is emotionally alone.

The Reality: How to Respond

As discussed earlier, emotional storms are predictable reactions to cancer. Anyone involved with that illness who does not experience such feelings as fear, anxiety, sadness, despair, or depression at times would be well advised to consult a therapist. Caregivers need not worry if the patient or they themselves feel many strong emotions. They need to worry only if they don't.

Trying to deny, suppress, or fight such feelings, or worrying about having them, is counterproductive. Emotions are natural responses to what is happening. As long as we acknowledge and in some way express them, they give us information about what is going on inside and outside ourselves that helps us to survive and to experience what life offers. When we avoid, resist, or hide them, they don't go away. Instead, they often just become distorted (Kübler-Ross, 1987). Keeping a stiff upper lip is often recommended, but often not very useful. The question is not whether to feel the emotions we have, but how to deal with them.

Myth #3: Cancer is an inevitable death sentence.

Regardless of what they might know to the contrary, many people regard cancer as an incurable disease usually leading to a slow, painful death. After a diagnosis, patients and family members, believing that the patient is doomed and helpless, often are more concerned about why the cancer occurred than about what they can do about it. They are unaware of the many ways that modern medicine can greatly improve the chances of recovery.

The Reality: How to Respond

Most people diagnosed with cancer do not die of it. Survival rates have increased dramatically over the years and continue to do so. As improved and new methods of prevention, diagnosis, and treatment are developed, more and more people can be expected to recover from all kinds of cancer. There is no form of cancer with a 100% mortality rate, no kind of cancer from which no one has ever recovered. Most cancers can be cured, and many others—including those that have spread beyond the original site—can be controlled for a long time with a succession of treatments.

Besides receiving medical treatment, patients themselves can do numerous things to make it more likely to recover or at least to extend their lives. As is discussed in Part II, there are many ways that family members can help to make this happen.

Myth #4: Medical statistics foretell the future.

Another deadly popular belief is that a physician who cites a bleak and terrifying statistical prognosis ("There is a 50% survival rate," "Life expectancy is 6 months to a year," "The most that can be expected is remission for a while") is a prophet predicting the future with 100% accuracy.

The Reality: How to Respond

Physicians are unable to predict any individual's life expectancy accurately, and many no longer try. Their prognostic forecasts are based on statistics about groups of people who were studied. Conclusions drawn from those research studies pertain to the people who were in those groups, not to anyone else. People included in such studies are often of a variety of ages, disease stages, and general physical and psychological health. Statistics gathered from these studies are about averages, not about any individual. For that reason, from the conclusions of those studies, it is not possible to make predictions about any individual. Physicians cannot know how a patient will respond to cancer and treatment. They cannot know the strength of that individual's immune system, or the ability of the person's mind and body to rally. Prognoses are simply odds—and are frequently defied. Many patients are not ready to die when their physicians think they are supposed to, and often they far outlive medical expectations. No one's future is determined by statistics drawn from groups of other people.

More than 25 years ago, long before many present-day treatments were developed, Dr. John MacDonald, a physician, wrote:

> Many cancers carry highly favorable prognoses. . . . Even the most unfavorable forms are highly unpredictable in their behavior. Besides, nearly every known form of cancer today has been associated with a prolonged remission or complete spontaneous regression. Even seemingly hopeless cancers have been cured. (1982, p. 61)

In short, the reality is that no one can know who will get well or how long anyone will live. It is not possible to assign a statistic to any individual's survival. Every health care practitioner has seen patients die suddenly when they had every medical reason to get well. They have also seen others get well whose medical outlook was hopeless. Patients can be sure that some people with the same kind of cancer as theirs might have died of it, that others lived a very long time after their diagnosis, and that some died of old age. No one can know which group any individual will be in. There is only one survival statistic that is absolutely, 100%, certain: the human death rate is one per person.

I had the good fortune to study with Anna Cassirer Appelbaum, the best psychotherapist I have ever encountered. At the time she was in her late 80s and still seeing patients and supervisees. She was very frail, with many physical problems, including a heart condition that she had had for many years. She told me that 35 years earlier her cardiologist had warned, "You have to quit work and go to bed. You could drop dead at any moment." "So could you, Doctor!" she replied. That cardiologist died not long afterward. Two that followed him also died. Anna died in her early 90s.

Suppose a doctor says that 50% of people with the same kind of cancer as the patient in question live for 5 years. This does not mean that in 5 years the patient will be 50% alive. In 5 years he will be either 100% alive or 100% dead—and which he will be cannot be predicted. While statistics drawn from studies are useful guidelines for physicians in recommending treatments, not even the most elaborate statistical calculations can predict how long anyone will live. The most truthful, accurate, and beneficial answer any doctor can give to the question, "How long do I have?" is "I don't know—and no one else knows either."

Patients need not be passive, helpless spectators in their healing process. They can change the statistics about their illness. When they actively pursue an integrated program—for example, medical treatment combined with an individualized nutritional program, along with psychotherapy or any other complementary treatments they feel are right for them—they are bringing to bear their body's own natural healing abilities. In so doing, they are changing the statistics, raising the odds in their favor.

To paraphrase my mentor and long-time colleague Lawrence Le-Shan, "Physicians who quote survival statistics often feel that they have to play God, but so few of them have the qualifications."

Patients and family members need to believe (if not always, then at least most of the time) and to be accorded the conviction that the person with cancer can get well, no matter what the odds (Siegel, 1998).

CHAPTER 5

The Power of Expectation

Hope deferred maketh the heart sick; but when the desire cometh, it is a tree of life.

Proverbs 13:12

Throughout the history of medicine, one main cause of healing probably has been patients' positive expectations, along with the body's ability for self-renewal. In his book *The Anatomy of Hope*, the physician Jerome Groopman said that for all his patients, hope has proved to be as important as any medication he might prescribe or any procedure he might perform. (2003, p. xiii)

From the first therapy session, besides trying to identify baseless beliefs, therapists need to learn about the patient's and family's expectations of recovery. Some families are, for the most part, hopeful that the person who is ill can fight for her life, beat any odds, and regain her health. Others are hopeless and remain so. If the family assumes that the patient is going to die, it is hard, if not impossible, for the patient to have hope and determination. Therapists, as well as doctors, can have a strong influence on these expectations. For this reason, this chapter discusses the power of expectation in some detail.

The 19th-century philosopher William James once remarked that there is no clear dividing line between a person's philosophy and physiology. Since the middle of the 20th century, modern mind-body research studies have confirmed his idea. They have found increasing evidence that recovery from illness can be strongly influenced by psychological and emotional factors. All the different aspects of a person interact and influence one another. While expectations do not determine outcomes, they can strengthen or weaken the powers of self-healing and recovery.

Negative expectation on the part of family members can be psychologically destabilizing and injurious, not only to the patient, but to everyone else in the family. For those family members, giving up might be a self-protective measure. Believing the situation is hopeless, they might try to distance themselves from the patient's emotional suffering. When they do, however, their attitude is readily communicated to the person who is ill (LeShan, 1980). If the patient expects to die soon and this belief persists, it may not only weaken her body's self-healing abilities but can lead to inaction that makes it a self-fulfilling prophecy.

If, on the other hand, regardless of even a bleak medical prognosis family members say that they will do everything to help fight for the patient's life, their determination and positive expectations are very likely to influence the patient's attitude, and possibly even the course of the illness.

Most people with cancer have some kind of expectation about the likelihood of their recovery. Their expectations are reflected in their emotional reactions to the illness and can play a significant part in their response to treatment and the chances of regaining their health. (In some major hospitals today, if a patient scheduled for elective surgery expresses the expectation belief that he will not survive, the surgery is cancelled.)

The power of expectation is illustrated clearly by a classic, frequently cited case reported in the early 1950s by a colleague of Dr. Bruno Klopfer, who documented it (1951, pp. 331–340). Although it is a single incident, it is difficult to discount. A patient, "Mr. Wright," had advanced widespread lymphosarcoma, a cancer of the lymph nodes, and was no longer responding to radiation. His body was riddled with tumors, some of which Dr. Klopfer described as being the size of oranges. All standard treatments had failed. The patient had to take oxygen through a mask and fluid had to be drained from his chest every few days. He was expected to live no more than a few weeks. A new experimental drug, Krebiozen, had been touted in the medical journals and then picked up by the newspapers as a potential miracle cure for cancer. Wright knew that his physician was involved in testing the drug and asked to get it. Although the doctor did not expect any response, at Wright's pleading, the doctor agreed to include him in the clinical trial. Shortly after he administered one injection of the drug, the patient's tumor masses, Klopfer wrote, "melted like snowballs on a hot stove," and in only a few days shrank drastically. Mr. Wright was soon released from the hospital, apparently free of malignancy, and resumed his normal life.

Then the press published reports from the AMA and the FDA that the drug was not as great an advance as had been believed. Wright's tumors returned quickly. Suspecting that this was due to his expectations, the doctor decided to use him as a control patient. He told Wright that he would give him a double-strength dose of a new, more active form of the drug—then injected him with distilled water. Again the tumors melted away. For the next 2 months Wright lived without symptoms, running his own business and flying his plane. Then the newspapers reported that, beyond a doubt, Krebiozen was found to be worthless. Wright appeared at the hospital a few days later. His tumors grew massive, and he died within two days.

A more common example of the powerful effects of expectation is found in patients treated with chemotherapy. Chemotherapy drugs often have negative side effects, but they can be made worse by the fact that patients sometimes feel sick before receiving the drugs, sometimes when they arrive at the treatment center or even the evening before. They involuntarily learn to get sick as a conditioned response. (It should be noted that such conditioned responses sometimes can be reversed.)

Numerous studies of the effects of placebos show clearly that our healing abilities are affected by our expectations. Placebos are inert substances containing no active ingredients, or physical or verbal procedures that the patient believes to have healing qualities. The substances might be, for example, sugar pills or the distilled water that was administered to Mr. Wright. Procedures might be diets, rituals, injections, psychological interventions, or physical touch. What they all have in common is that the subject believes in their power to heal. Researchers report that placebos have been found to help many kinds of medical conditions, including breathing problems, hay fever, coughs, skin conditions, fevers, headaches, wound pains, hay fever, seasickness, arthritis, hypertension, and peptic ulcers. They can also affect such processes as white blood cell count and respiratory rates and can change body chemistry. Placebos can also have negative effects, including nausea, weakness, or pain. Such effects are not just imagined. Actual physical changes have often been observed and measured. Modern trials of new drugs almost always include the use of a placebo. Neither the researchers nor the subjects know which patients being tested are receiving a placebo in place of the actual drug. At times patients have responded as well to the placebo as to the drug. (It needs to be noted here that this is not done in trials with cancer drugs, where use of a placebo would be unethical. In this case, one group of cancer patients receives standard chemotherapy drugs while the other receives the same drugs plus the one being tested.)

About placebos used in drug studies, R. Delap, one of the physicians heading the U.S. Food and Drug Administration's Offices of Drug Evaluation, said that expectation is a powerful thing: the more you believe you will benefit from a treatment, the more likely it is that you will experience a benefit (quoted in Nordenberg, 2000).

In a study about women and aging, researchers predictably found that as a rule, women who followed nutritional guidelines and exercised regularly lived longer. Less predictable was the finding that another factor also contributed to their longevity: their positive expectations. Elderly women who had expected to continue to be well, energetic, and vital as they aged lived nearly a decade longer than those who expected to become increasingly debilitated. Researchers in various countries have reported that optimistic people tend to live longer than pessimists (Holt, 2007). Perhaps, as has been speculated, optimism confers a survival advantage by helping people cope with adversity.

Expectations of cancer patients and their families about being well do not arise simply out of the patient's felt physical condition and the medical prognosis. At least two other factors are involved.

One is a long-standing underlying metaphysical belief about how the world works, a belief that shapes the attitude with which people habitually approach life. People who believe that they cannot have an effect on what happens to them react to illness with the same helplessness they learned early in life. Believing that life disappoints them no matter what they do, they respond to the diagnosis in their habitual way, with their habitual negativity, catastrophic thinking, depression, and immobilization. Those who believe that good things happen or that they can have some control over adversity are more likely to decide that the family's fight against cancer can be won.

Besides habitual optimistic or pessimistic ways of thinking, another factor affecting families' expectations is the attitude of their health professionals. Patients' belief about the effectiveness of medical procedures can have an effect on how well those procedures work—and their practitioners affect those expectations.

Psychiatrist Jerome Frank wrote, "Physicians have known that their ability to inspire expectant trust in a patient partially determines the success of the treatment" (1991, p. 133). Bernie Siegel said, "A patient's confidence in a certain treatment can be negated by the doctor's unspoken rejection of it" (1998, p. 37). Dutch psychiatrist Marco DeVries, who specialized in work with cancer patients, made the same point:

> The [health professional] himself becomes an important factor in the healing process, a factor which may have a favorable and sadly, in certain circumstances, an unfavorable effect on the process. . . . The healing process may be influenced not only by the

patient's frame of mind, but also by the physician's views and ideas on disease, his expectations and his motives. (1993, p. 94)

The power of belief extends far beyond the effects of medication. Dr. Walter Cannon, who identified the fight-or-flight response, observed hospital patients from primitive societies who claimed to be hexed and watched them die of no cause he could determine. He discovered that in some cultures one human being can point at another human being, proclaim that at a specific time the person will die—and the prediction is fulfilled. These people accepted the "truth" of the witch doctor's prediction, and that "truth" led to death. The will to die replaces the will to live, and the individual accepts an appointment with death. As Norman Cousins, who did research in the biochemistry of human emotions, once put it, "their belief becomes their biology" (1989).

If an oncologist or surgeon delivers a diagnosis as if it were a death sentence, everyone in the family will be far more likely to respond accordingly. When a diagnostician paints a dismal or a worst-case picture ominously reinforced with statistics, or when a doctor says, "There is nothing more we can do" or predicts how long a patient will live, the curse will do its work. A patient given a 50% chance of living for 5 years interprets this as a 50% chance of dying. Probably everyone in the medical field has seen patients who accepted the truth of the doctor's prediction, and, like the accursed individual in a primitive society, complied on time (Dossey, 1992). Even if the practitioner's pessimism is communicated indirectly, the patient's health can be negatively affected. Similarly, when a psychotherapist is unconvinced that the patient can get better, even if that attitude is not expressed verbally, it is communicated, and the client knows it and is strongly affected by it.

If we can sentence ourselves to death and keep that appointment, we can often keep an appointment with life. If the mind can program the body to die, it can also program the body to live. While emotions do not cause cancer, they can sometimes affect its course in positive or negative ways. The feeling of helplessness, leading to negative expectations and hopelessness, is in itself a serious disease. "Nothing about cancer is more lethal than hopelessness and nothing is more essential than the determination to get the best out of whatever is possible" (Cousins, 1990, p. xvi).

Practitioners' words, beliefs, and even unspoken attitudes have enormous power to affect the lives of their clients. How can patients and family members have hope if their health practitioners convey hopelessness?

Any therapist working with clients dealing with cancer can expect to hear stories about physicians who have devastated patients and their families with a dire prognosis. The clients' resulting fear and despair then become a major issue for therapy. Physicians are often concerned not to give what is usually called false hope, but what does false hope mean? It means that the person who is sick cannot get better, so that there is no reason for hope. This concept of false hope apparently is intended to prevent disappointment. However, it also prevents any incentive for living as fully as possible, or for dealing actively with an illness that threatens life. No one can possibly know that any individual cannot get better. We can know with certainty that someone was dying only after the person is dead. This belief, that the patient is doomed and that there is no realistic stance other than pessimism can serve only to further a negative outcome.

Rather than false hope, it would be more reasonable to think in terms of "false hopelessness" or "false doom." There is always reason for hope. One of the main tasks of any psychotherapist who works with clients dealing with cancer is to make it very clear to them that hope carries with it its own justification, so that it is always reasonable.

Since there is little dispute these days about the psychological and physical value of hope, a more accurate term would be *false expectations*. Physicians are concerned that if they do not tell the truth about a patient's condition, they will be lying. Of course any irresponsible information or advice—whether it is about conventional medical treatments, complementary treatments, psychological interventions, diets, or unproven remedies—can give rise to unrealistic expectations. For that reason physicians tend to be conservative in their claims. Unfortunately patients and family members invariably hear this as pure pessimism, for which they pay a high price (Cunningham, 2005). The fundamental principle of medical ethics is the Hippocratic dictum, "Above all, do no harm." Health practitioners of all kinds working with people trying to cope with cancer need to understand that this kind of pessimism is likely to do psychological harm (Bolletino, 1998).

The most helpful practitioners are those who do not allow statistics to determine their attitude, words, and behavior. There are ways and ways of saying anything. From those clients fortunate enough to have physicians who know that their own outlook can affect the lives of the people in their care, I have learned that it is possible to convey and discuss even the most alarming information so that the patients respond with hope and determination, as with any challenge. When this happens, the person's body might also respond.

Janet, who had completed treatment for ovarian cancer a year earlier, was found to have a recurrence. A laparoscopy revealed numerous widespread small tumors as well as a larger inoperable tumor. Her surgeon had minimized these findings to her, and it was up to the oncologist to tell her and her family members the whole story. He said, "We found small cancer cells in your peritoneal area, as well as a 2 centimeter tumor on your spleen. I understand that this sounds frightening, but I want you to know that I am not about to dig a hole and bury you. No one is giving up. There are treatments that can be used that have been effective. Here is what I propose we do . . ." While giving an accurate and complete report, this physician acknowledged his patient's fear and also conveyed hope. With his word *we* he let her know that she was not alone, that there were people working for her health. She said that since she and her husband left his office, for the first time in weeks they both felt optimistic and energized, ready to do whatever it took to beat her disease.

All patients and their families need to be to be reassured that everything possible will be done, that they will not be abandoned by any of their practitioners, and that treatments are available. One of the most important things mental health professionals can do for their clients is to instill and encourage hope, no matter what the medical situation. Hope is not denial, delusion, or the groundless conviction that everything will be fine no matter what the situation. Hope is the recognition of the situation coupled with information about the path most likely to be effective. It is the realization that healing and recovery are possible, along with the determination to take steps to try to make that happen.

What is the problem with hope when no one can really know what will happen? It is important that patients and families always remember that there is no kind of cancer from which no one has ever recovered, and that it is not unusual for remissions to occur that are inexplicable from a medical viewpoint. Untold numbers of cancer patients diagnosed with "incurable" cancers have recovered with the help of medical doctors, appropriate treatments, and their own determination. Even if someone had a kind of cancer from which 9 out of 10 people have died, what would be the problem with her believing that she might be the 10th? What would be the problem with therapists encouraging their clients to believe that, too? Family members and patients need to understand that recovery is possible, and also to know that their practitioners are convinced of it.

For some people, though, hope feels risky.

I remember Sarah, who was in treatment for ovarian cancer. She once said, "Sometimes lately I start to feel hopeful, but I'm afraid to."

"Afraid why?" I asked.

"Because," she said, "I might be wrong."

After thinking this over, I said, "Well then, what are you afraid of? What's the worst that can happen? That you'll die and then feel like a fool?"

Like Sarah, many people are afraid to hope. They don't want to risk being disappointed or wrong. Hope might seem dangerous for other reasons as well.

Bruce, whose wife, Debby, was dealing with lung cancer, also expressed his fear of allowing himself hope. When I asked why, particularly since Debby was responding well to treatment, he admitted that he was afraid he might jinx her survival by expecting her to get well. I had to point out to him that even if he were to set out deliberately to jinx her recovery, hope would be unlikely to accomplish that.

Hopelessness carries with it other problems. It can prevent good treatment decisions when only the negative side of each treatment option is seen. It can prevent confidence about treatments, and make it harder to deal with discomfort. In the face of uncertainty, nothing is wrong with hope. It is by far the better of the two alternatives.

From time to time I hear from another former client, Anne, who sends family pictures and tells me what she, her husband Burt, and their children have been up to lately. At the time of this writing, it is 9 years since Burt was found to have a stage IV brain tumor, regarded by all his physicians as being impossible to survive. For at least 9 years, his tests have shown no trace of cancer.

Therapists and other health professionals often underrate the power of their words and even their unspoken attitudes and beliefs in the lives of people dealing with cancer. Practitioners' negative expectation that there is nothing to be done to help a patient recover can confirm the family's worst fears and impede the patient's healing process. Pessimism is intertwined with depression, and depression is linked with impaired immune function. As long as optimism does not prevent them from seeking the best possible treatment, people dealing with cancer must be accorded the belief that the patient might get well, no matter what the odds, and that without a doubt the fight is worth-while. After all, optimists are known to live longer, healthier lives than pessimists, even when pessimists might have a more accurate (so-called realistic) sense of the situation.

Information is therapeutic and necessary for hope. Negative beliefs and expectations can be changed once clients become aware of the ones they hold and of their effects. Therapists can guide clients into recognizing these beliefs. They can teach them to understand that statistics and pronouncements about survival time do not represent the word of God. They can furnish accurate information about how cancer develops and how treatments work. (Appendixes 1, 2, and 3 provide such information.) They can explain that patients need not be passive and powerless in the healing process, for there is much that they themselves can do to help themselves get better. They need to point out that there are people who have recovered from just about every known form of cancer, and so why shouldn't the patient in the client's family be one of them? Whether or not the patient's physicians do this, it is surely an important part of the psychotherapists' task.

In the Second World War the Allied armies taught soldiers in the Special Forces who were going behind enemy lines, "Never give up until you're caught." Similarly, it becomes part of effective psychotherapy with caregivers to teach them to instruct the patients they care for, "Never give up until you're sure that you're dead." After years of mind-body research, there is no longer a question as to whether psychological factors can affect the course of cancer and treatment. The only question is how to best direct those factors to mobilize the body's self-healing abilities.

CHAPTER 6

Dealing With Feelings

The human heart is like a ship on a stormy sea driven about by winds blowing from all four corners of heaven.

Martin Luther, Introduction to the *Psalms*

Family members, like the patients they are caring for, feel they have been flung suddenly into an alien world where they don't know the rules, and the rules shift constantly. Stress is almost constant as they try to deal with their fears and anxiety, with the effects of the illness and treatment on the patient and on themselves, and with a constant onslaught of responsibilities: medical appointments, nursing, housework, paperwork, long hours, and the outpouring of dollars. Family interactions as well as roles and responsibilities change when someone becomes ill, and perhaps incapacitated and more dependent, perhaps also more withdrawn or demanding.

For the sake of the person who is ill, family members try to remain outwardly cheerful, optimistic, and supportive. Inwardly, they are in turmoil and despair. Their emotions are just as bewildering and destabilizing to them as their situation. The emotional drain and their resulting fatigue is often enormous. While everyone's experience is different, one husband, who had cared for his wife for years, described his experience as "an unrelenting progression of exhaustion, anger, isolation, and resentment, mixed with the guilt that one should not have these feelings about someone you love but whose condition has nevertheless bound you in a daily emotional prison" (Wolpe, 2000, p. 39). As a result of all this, often family caregivers' sense of self and of their place in the world can erode.

In therapy, one step toward reestablishing their sense of self is for family members to bring their confused emotions to the surface to be discussed and sorted out. When they are able to state how they feel, and what they want and need, they begin to regain their awareness of who they are. Acknowledging and expressing their emotions clarifies them. It dissolves the stress of holding them in, and makes those feelings less frightening and overwhelming (Fiore, 1990). It also makes them easier to change.

Yet, just at this time when expression and clarity can be so important for them, many caregivers, like patients, often feel that they should not be having the feelings they do, let alone putting words to them. Some inhibit their emotions, often to try to shelter the patient, other family members, or friends. Some caregivers cannot bring themselves to discuss their situation or even to react fully. Even though at times they might feel helpless, desperate, sad, angry, frustrated, lonely, hopeless, and confused, they often believe that they would not be handling their situation well if they were to be anything but unfailingly composed, optimistic, tolerant, understanding, and loving. Many feel that asking for help indicates weakness.

This chapter discusses ways therapists can help caregivers deal with their emotional distress. While there is far more to psychotherapy with these clients than encouraging emotional expression, this kind of work is often a necessary place to begin.

Telling the Story

Our innumerable actions, small and large, write the narrative of our lives, which in turn describes us. The narrative is not only an assemblage of empirical facts; it is an aesthetic whole—a tapestry woven from individual threads to form a coherent pattern that is complete in itself, but that also tells of the weaver. (Cassell, 1994, p. 166)

Everyone has a story, "a narrative of their life." When we recount that story in therapy, what we choose to tell is what we consider most important. Shortly after any traumatic situation, we might need to tell our story, even again and again. The way we tell it expresses a great deal about who we are. We need to relate not only what has happened, but our thoughts and feelings about it. Sometimes imparting our own account of what happened is more important to us than describing or venting our feelings about it.

Eva, a divorced mother of two, called me for an appointment after her 20-year-old son Don had surgery for colon cancer and was in the middle of a course of radiation treatments. She began our first session by reciting the medical history of Don's situation, replete with technical terms: his initial symptoms, the physicians and specialists consulted, the tests taken, the test results, the formal diagnosis, the surgery, the surgeons' findings, and their conclusions. I listened, waiting for a more personal account, but in a tight, flat, wooden tone, she offered only a careful, formal, organized report. She looked as if she was concentrating on remembering all the factual details and technical terms and presenting them accurately, as if she was delivering a script she had prepared and practiced. In a way that is exactly what she was doing. In the family's frantic search for a cure, Eva had spent many evenings researching Don's kind of cancer and treatments on the Internet and had talked to a number of medical specialists.

It was clear that she needed to tell her story, but just as clear that the technical facts she recited were serving to distance her from her experience and her feelings. "Eva," I said after a while, "I'm not a physician. You don't need to explain all these technical details for me. I understand the diagnosis and the treatments. What's been happening to Don is terrible for him. How has all this been for you?"

Her face lost its tight composure. She sagged into the couch and, like a lost child, began to cry. "It's been hard. So hard . . ."

After a few moments, I asked quietly, "What's been the hardest part?"

She no longer edited her words and just let them pour out. "He's so young and so sick. He has so much to live for. He's been so brave. And he has more surgery ahead of him, awful surgery. This shouldn't be happening to him. It should never have happened. I hate seeing him this way. The doctors can't make any promises. I'm so afraid he'll die, and I can't let him know that. I don't ever want him to know how terrified I am and how hard it is to see him going through this."

She wept, she talked, and I listened intently. Now, instead of a medical history, she told her personal story, beginning with how she and Don learned about the diagnosis and how they reacted. As the session went on, she became increasingly open, her voice became stronger, and she seemed far more relaxed.

At the end of our time together, before she got up to leave, she wiped her eyes, took out a mirror, put on lipstick, and patted down her hair. After rearranging herself so that she looked as she did when she arrived, she left, better armed against her situation and all that she had to face.

Like many caregivers, Eva was concerned not to upset the person who was ill by revealing her fears, her grief, her feelings of helplessness, and her anxiety. She said that unless she showed only a calm, cheerful facade, she would burden him, take away his hope, and cause him more fear and suffering.

There are other reasons caregivers might give themselves for keeping their emotions at bay:

- "I hate feeling this way. It feels awful."
- "I shouldn't be feeling this way."
- "I'm ashamed of some of my feelings."
- "She is suffering so much more than I am. She needs me to stay strong."
- "If I don't keep a stiff upper lip, I might get really depressed."
- "When I start thinking about how bad I feel, I feel selfish and guilty."
- "If I let myself feel all those emotions that keep coming up, I'll just cave in and won't be able to do all the things I have to take care of."
- "I just don't have the time to be concerned about all my feelings."
- "I don't want to be weak."
- "If I let myself be afraid, people will think I'm weak."
- "If I start to cry, I won't be able to stop."
- "If I talk about how awful this situation is, people will think I'm just feeling sorry for myself."
- "What right do I have to feel sorry for myself when the person I love is so sick, and suffering so much?"
- "How can I get angry at him when he is so sick?"
- "I can't tell her how I feel because she might just break down and start to cry, and I wouldn't know what to do then."

For one reason or another, many caregivers believe not only that they should stifle their feelings, but that they shouldn't be feeling what they do. They judge some emotions to be wrong, even shameful. They might regard them as being less important than those of the person who is ill, and think that paying attention to what they are feeling would be selfish. As a result, they might not talk to anyone about what they feel.

Even if they want to talk, often they feel that there is no one to talk to who can listen and understand. Sometimes they find that if they try to express what their experience is like, others can't or don't want to hear them. It is not unusual for people involved with cancer to discover that even some people close to them might avoid them. It is often difficult for others to listen or even to be with them because they find it painful or uncomfortable. However much they care, they might not know how to help or even to react. Listening might trigger their own fears, reminding them of their own vulnerability and mortality.

Al, who had been caring for his wife, Cindy, since her diagnosis of ovarian cancer 6 months earlier, said, "I've been handling everything in the house, and trying my best to give Cindy the love and support she needs. I'm lucky I work for myself so I can set up my work schedule. I want to help in any way I can, with the house, the kids, and anything she needs. At least it's doing something. My mother-in-law came to stay with us to help out for a month, and Cindy's sisters took turns coming here for a while, too. Cindy's had a lot of bad reactions to her treatments, or maybe it's to the cancer. Some days she has to spend almost all the time in bed. Lately she's been very weak, and sometimes in pain. It's been so hard for her that I try not to think about my own feelings.

"I tell myself that compared to what she's going through, I have it easy. But sometimes it gets to be too much. She's not getting better, and I'm getting more afraid. I think I might be acting weird sometimes. I have to be a husband and a father, to stay strong for her and the kids and everyone else, but it's getting harder and harder. When she gets upset I hold her and say, 'It'll all be all right, baby. You'll be all right.' . . . But sometimes . . . sometimes I just can't be the strong guy. I can't talk to Cindy's mother or sisters about how it is for me, because they're going through such a hard time, too. It's awful for them to see her like this and know they might lose her. They've come to me and cried.

"So when one of Cindy's sisters was staying with us, I went out to be with some old buddies of mine. We've been friends since we went to high school. When they asked me how things were, I found myself really telling them what was going on and how I was feeling. I had to. I couldn't keep it all in anymore. There was no one else I could talk to. They had never heard me talk that way, and they seemed surprised, but they were great. They said they didn't know that things were that bad. I felt a lot better, so much relief letting it all out. I saw them again a couple weeks later and they asked how things were going. So I started to tell them, but after a while they didn't want to listen anymore. I guess I was telling them more than they bargained for, more than they wanted to hear. They tried to cheer me up. They offered me a drink. They changed the subject. When I saw them again a couple days ago, they asked about how Cindy was, but I could tell they didn't really want to know a lot about it. I guess it was hard for them to listen. Maybe after hearing it before, it got boring or depressing, or maybe I got boring or depressing, or maybe I scared them and they just didn't know what to say."

When, for whatever reason, caregivers hold it all in, their feelings intensify and sometimes come out in ways they don't intend. When they come to therapy, their first need is to tell their story—not the kind of precise clinical report they give to doctors, but the story of their personal experiences, whatever form that takes.

As the patient's medical situation changes, neither the caregivers' emotions nor their need to talk abates.

Like Eva, who began her first therapy session with a detailed recitation of medical facts, the client might start with a clinical account: the patient's symptoms, the diagnosis, the treatment, and, very likely, the statistical prognosis. To be sure, therapists need to know about the patient's medical situation, but what is far more important at this point is that the client be encouraged to tell her own story. The therapist can do this with just a few words. ("Tell me, how has this been for you?" "What's been the hardest part?" "What were you thinking and feeling when you learned the diagnosis?")

Shortly after any traumatic situation, people usually need to tell their story, sometimes again and again. However they tell it, they should never be pressured to say more than what they are naturally inclined to. If the client does not want to relive her experience and describe it in detail, it might be because she is not ready to do so, or because she is putting her pain on hold until she has more strength or a clearer perspective. Whatever way family members talk about their personal experiences is the right way for them to do so. The therapist would do well to invite them to say more, but that is all. Whatever the story, what is important is that it is told, that it is a meaningful story to the client, and that it is heard and understood.

More Than One Story to Tell

Every loss in a person's life is connected to every other. Caregivers who have experienced losses in the past may well have a particularly difficult time dealing with their present situation.

> From the time of Jason's diagnosis of a malignant brain tumor, his wife, Kathy, was supportive to him in every possible way while she herself remained confident about his recovery. For over a year Jason's physicians regarded him as a star patient: he responded well to his treatments, experienced minimal side effects, continued to feel strong and energetic, and even began working out at a gym. ("It's hard for me to believe that anything is wrong with me," he would say with a grin.) Then test results showed that the tumor was growing again. Within only a few months he spent more and more time sleeping, his affect became flat, and he lost his short-term memory. For the first time since the diagnosis, Kathy caved in. "It's horrible for me to be with him now. He's been getting worse and worse, and now he doesn't even remember what happened an hour ago. He reminds me every day of those years I took care of care of my dad when he had Alzheimer's."

Kathy had two stories she needed to tell. Her experiences had to be differentiated and separated, for her reactions to Jason's cancer were mixed with her experiences with her father. In this situation we had to go back to the past. She talked about her father, his decline, his death, and how she felt throughout the various stages of his ordeal. After that story, such questions as these helped to begin clarifying the present:

- "How was your experience with your dad the same as what's happening now with Jason?"
- "How was it different?"
- "How were the feelings you had with your dad the same as what you're feeling now with Jason?"
- "How were they different?"

How to Listen

Most people dealing with cancer need to talk and be heard by someone willing to listen and to experience the pain they express (Kane, 2003). Telling their story can help them let in its reality (Hope, 2005). Recounting it again (and even again) can help them believe it and can lessen their pain. When they talk, they need to feel that what they say is received and understood by someone listening with calm concern. To the extent that they are heard and met in this way, their anxiety lessens and they can speak more openly.

Many clients in therapy who are not dealing with a life-threatening illness expect their therapists to fix them: to solve their problems or take away their pain. This usually is not the case with family caregivers or people with cancer. They don't expect to be fixed. What they do need is to be heard, seen, and understood. At this point in the therapy, the therapist's only appropriate response is just to listen to the clients' story and to what their experiences mean to them. Questions and even encouraging words might be out of place.

The focus is not on looking for psychological symptoms or a diagnosis, and there is nothing to be interpreted or analyzed. *The only valid interpretations and analyses are the client's own, for it is the client, not the therapist, who is the authority on herself.* At this point, most of all these clients need their suffering understood and acknowledged. Only in this way can it be lessened. What this means is that the traditional professional stance of objectivity is unhelpful, as are traditional techniques. Like most people in crisis who are raw and vulnerable, these clients have a built-in detector for inauthenticity and are likely to react to therapeutic techniques as being false, hollow, or even manipulative.

The therapist needs to listen openly, receptively, with deep interest and complete attention. Everything about the story and the way it is related—the words used, the body language, the pitch, the tone, tempo, and intensity—conveys something about the speaker. This is not the time to take notes, to make judgments, or to think in terms of symptoms, problems, or diagnostic labels. Listening this way entails focusing to get a sense of the individual as a complex human being and what he is experiencing. It entails only being and feeling with the other with compassion, not just trying to figure the person out. Only in this way can the therapist enter accurately into the client's world. (The word *compassion* means "feeling" or "suffering with." It does not mean "pity" or "being separate from.")

It is very possible that at some point early on these clients will express embarrassment, guilt, or shame, perhaps for being annoyed, resentful, or overwhelmed with all they have to handle, and for wishing that the situation would just end. They need to understand that as intense and tumultuous as their feelings may be, they are natural reactions to the crisis in their lives. They need to learn not to judge any of their feelings, whatever they are. Therapists can legitimize these clients' emotions by explaining their normalcy.

Accepting Emotions: A Lecture for Clients

Emotions are often described and classified as being either positive or negative. People often judge them as acceptable or unacceptable, appropriate or inappropriate, mature or childish.

These classifications are unhelpful. Emotions may be pleasant or unpleasant, but they aren't positive or negative, good or bad. They aren't logical. They just are. We don't choose what we feel. We can't decide to feel some emotions (the so-called positive ones that we like) and not others (the ones we call negative that we don't like). Even if we are able to disavow emotions we don't want, maybe because we believe they are unacceptable, dangerous, or unpleasant, we pay a high price. If we don't express or at least acknowledge them, they gnaw at us and affect us emotionally and physically.

There are different, more productive ways to look at emotions than as positive or negative. Feelings like fear, anger, grief, and depression can be seen instead as natural symptoms of cancer and treatment that can be expected from time to time. They are normal, healthy, predictable reactions to a terrible situation.

A useful classification of emotions is the one used by Elisabeth Kübler-Ross. Rather than positive or negative, she regarded them as being either natural or distorted (Bolletino, 1996).

Natural emotions—anger, fear, grief, and love—are those for which we human beings have an innate capacity. They are our responses to our inner and outer environments. So long as such emotions are acknowledged and in some way expressed or dealt with, they provide information that aids survival and helps us experience what life offers. When we repress our natural emotions, they fester and become distorted. In that form they can easily become displaced almost at random in all directions and projected out into the world. Disowning emotions does not cause them to disappear. It only causes us to be unable to act on them in ways we choose.

Cancer brings with it many reasons for anger. Anger is a natural emotion and an honorable one. It mobilizes us to try to bring about change. It enables us to assert and to protect ourselves. It helps us to define our selves and our boundaries by reflecting what we don't want. It can take the form of moral passion that impels us to act to protect our integrity, our principles, our lives, or the lives of others.

Unacknowledged or unexpressed, anger distorts. At the very least we might withdraw, becoming uncommunicative and morose. Instead we might lash out, usually at the people closest to us, or simply deny how we feel, pretending to ourselves and others that we aren't angry at all. When we deal with anger in any of these ways, it just smolders, creating physical tension and emotional stress. It distorts. Repressed anger can distort into resentment, a desire for revenge, bitterness, hatred of other people and of the self, or rage. It can also manifest as hostility, powerlessness, violence, suicide, or depression. When, instead of withdrawing, lashing out, or denying anger, we can acknowledge it, feel it, and articulate or express it in some benign way, it ends. Consider, for example, small children playing together. One might grab a toy from the other. They might shriek angrily, even hit each other—and then it's over. Their anger is out and then gone, and they play peaceably together again.

Fear is another natural emotion. It protects us, alerting us to danger so that we are ready in an instant to fight or flee. Without it we could not survive. Repressed, it can become distorted and turn into anxiety, panic, irrational prejudice, psychosomatic pain, phobias, dread of the future, hostile rage, or even acts of violence. Too often people believe that expressing or even feeling fear is a sign of weakness. In fact, just the opposite is true. When we express fear we often feel stronger. For example, expressing the fear that the patient whom we love might not survive can sometimes turn that fear around or lessen it.

Grief is a natural emotion. It is the normal reaction to loss and separation. With cancer we experience loss in every part our life. When we can let ourselves feel grief, experience it, and express it, it softens and sooner or later ends. When we resist it and don't deal with our losses, grief can distort into self-pity, bitterness, chronic depression or anxiety, and never end (Bolletino, 1996).

Emotions are often experienced as physical feelings. When we habitually deny emotions, smother them, or learn to distract ourselves from them, we can become physically as well as psychically numb, barely aware of what we feel in our bodies at all. However, the feelings don't disappear, and we might be courting severe physical reactions. One man, who described himself as "a caregiver without training" for his wife, wrote in an article, "Recently I realized that . . . I had turned emotionally inward in an attempt to maintain control. I banked many of my emotions in the name of efficiency. I internalized my own sorrow, anger, frustration and fear for the sake of my wife who was battling her own inner struggles." It took its toll, he added: within a few years he had a heart attack (Wolpe, 2000, p. 37).

In short, contrary to the widespread belief that we should always be serene, chirpy, and upbeat by stuffing our natural feelings inside us and keeping a stiff upper lip, in a situation like a life-threatening illness this does not help in any way. It can make us feel worse, if only because it takes up a lot of energy that would be better used in other ways.

Anyone caring for a family member with cancer needs to learn to have as much acceptance, tolerance, and compassion for their own feelings as they do for the emotions of the person who is ill. Feelings are not positive or negative, appropriate or inappropriate, good or bad, acceptable or unacceptable. They just are what they are. Usually they are just normal responses to what is happening. Since we can't choose them, it makes no sense to judge them. We can, however, choose what we do in response.

The surest way to deal with grief, anger, fear, and even despair, is to go right through the middle of these emotions. First, just acknowledge them, allow them, and accept them. Let it be all right that you feel them. Lean into them. After all, they are part of you at the moment, but they are not who you are. Then express them and go on feeling. If you do that, you will find that they moderate, soften, and pass. Then there is room for other emotions, like hope, excitement, and joy.

Marcel Proust knew this well when, in *Remembrance of Things Past*, he wrote, "We are healed of a suffering only by experiencing it to the fullest"

Dealing with Feelings

The therapist's response to caregivers' feelings can teach these clients an attitude toward themselves as well as toward the cancer patient. Family caregivers need to have their feelings encouraged, understood, accepted, and validated, not soothed. (For example, instead of, "That's unlikely to happen. There's no need to be frightened," it is far more helpful for the client to hear, "Yes, that must be very frightening. Do you want to say more about it?") Reassuring the patient might reduce the therapist's anxiety but does not help the client.

Expressing emotions as fully as possible often lessens them and can be a vital part of therapy with anyone dealing with cancer. Therapists who are not at ease with intense feelings (their own and those of others) would do well to think carefully about working with anyone dealing with cancer. Sooner or later they are guaranteed to push every one of the therapists' own emotional buttons.

Anxiety and Fear

I, a stranger and afraid
In a world I never made.

A. E. Housman,
Last Poems, #12

Family members might feel anxious whenever they think about the death of the person who is ill or about their own death, and at times they will be unable to stop themselves from thinking such thoughts. As a result they might have an overall feeling of apprehension that can be overwhelming, without being able to identify the exact danger or threat that they fear. They might just feel that something terrible is going to happen, and they don't know what.

Many people are afraid to feel fear. They are afraid of being afraid. When they try to deny and suppress their fears, the fears just intensify and become a kind of amorphous anxiety. Suppressing fear, as well as other emotions, not only uses energy but can also result in inadequate sleep, which only increases anxiety and also can lead to other emotional and physical symptoms.

Anxiety can be eased when the client can bring to light and admit each fear, one by one, and identify its cause. Because cancer is not fully understood and its course is not predictable, it brings with it many different fears that might or might not be well founded. Among the greatest ones is that the patient will die. This fear is increased if family members imagine a painful lingering death. They might feel fear if the patient isn't feeling better or getting better. They might fear medical treatments and procedures, and their side effects. A cancer diagnosis of someone they love might cause them to be fearful about their own health, wondering if they have or can get cancer, too. (It is not unusual for family members to start tracing their own medical genealogy at this time.) They also often fear what will happen to them if the patient dies and wonder how they can manage or even live without that person.

Each fear that is acknowledged needs to be clarified and explored. ("What do you think is going to happen?" "What frightens you about that?" "What's the worst thing that can happen?") Some fears can be dissolved simply with knowledge, since they are based on false assumptions, erroneous information, or past experiences that have no bearing on the present situation. Others—including the fear of death—can at least be lessened by being faced, expressed, clarified, and discussed.

Particularly in frightening, unpredictable situations, people can readily engage in catastrophic fantasies that build their anxiety. They imagine the worst possible scenarios and then regard them as the most likely. When this becomes apparent in therapy, it can be extremely helpful for clients to be made aware of what they are doing. Once this tendency is identified, explained, and labeled ("You're catastrophizing"), most clients can learn to become self-aware when they engage in this kind of destructive thinking and bring themselves back to the reality of the present.

The reality is that we do not know what is going to happen. Physician Jeff Kane, who facilitates cancer support groups, wrote that there are only four things we can know about someone who is sick and that she can know about herself:

1. We know she's sick.
2. We know that sick or not, she'll die: sick or not, she's as mortal as anyone else.
3. We know she's alive now.
4. We know our feelings as we relate to her. (2003, p. 129)

Denial

Nature never deceives us; it is we who deceive ourselves.

Rousseau, *Emile*

Denial comes and goes. At the outset it is a healthy mechanism to cope with the reality of cancer, and everyone in the family needs to retain as much of it as is necessary, as long as necessary, for their emotional survival. It might be the only way they can deal with the situation initially and at other times.

If it persists, however, it can lead to both practical and emotional problems. One major practical problem is that family members in denial about a patient's illness might not take the steps for treatment that could save the person's life. They might not make practical or legal arrangements, such as plans for home or hospice care, or for a living will, power of attorney, or trust funds. They are also unlikely to discuss what the patient wants by way of funeral arrangements, or to make legal arrangements that could help both the patient and themselves. (See Appendix 5 for legal options.)

Persistent denial can also isolate family members emotionally from one another. If either the patient or a family member denies the reality of what is happening ("Everything is going to be all right"), the other is alone, unable to discuss what is on his mind.

It is likely that those clients who persist in denying that cancer is a serious threat will also deny their feelings, surely their anger and depression, as they have probably done for most of their lives.

It is not helpful for the therapist to attempt to force clients to face emotions or dreaded possibilities they are not yet ready to deal with. For most people, however, there comes a time when denial can no longer be sustained. ("The diagnosis isn't a mistake." "I didn't even know how angry I am.")

There is an important difference between denial and hope. Denial is the refusal or inability to believe the reality of what is happening. It can take the form of the unrealistic optimistic conviction that no matter what the situation, everything will be fine. Hope, on the other hand, is the belief that whatever the present situation, there is a chance that things can change for the better. Family members and patients who believe in this possibility and maintain that they will do everything to fight for the patient's life, no matter what the odds, should be cheered on, not discouraged. This attitude can make a difference not only to their quality of life but to the patient's response to treatment.

Diana, whose husband, Jake, had cancer, said, "I try to tell myself that everything is going to be all right, that he is going to be well, but I don't always believe it."

I said, "Well, how about telling yourself what you really know: that he *might* get well. That's true, and you had better believe it. No one can know for sure, but it is certainly a possibility, and one worth fighting for. You and he are doing all that you can to make that happen, and you're doing a great job."

Anger and Resentment

I was angry with my friend;
I told my wrath, my wrath did end.

I was angry with my foe;
I told it not, my wrath did grow
William Blake, "The Poison Tree,"
Songs of Experience

There is no reason for family caregivers not to feel resentment and anger: at their loss of freedom and time for themselves, at all their new burdens, at mounting financial pressures, at feeling trapped, at the patient's dependence on them and lack of awareness and appreciation for all that they do, and, most of all, at the possibility that the patient might die and leave them. In view of all their efforts, they are likely to resent the patient's resentment toward them. (People with cancer, often angry at their dependence, their illness, and possible death, might direct it toward those closest to them.)

The underlying cause of caregivers' resentment and anger, however, usually is not the patient but the illness or the disability, and the unfairness of it. Losses make us angry. We often feel that the contract we made with the universe has been broken, so we feel cheated. Any close family member of someone with cancer has had numerous losses, certainly including the lives they had, the healthy person they knew, and the time and pleasures they had.

It is particularly helpful that clients be encouraged to give voice to their anger and resentments. ("You have no choices about what you feel, but you can choose what to do with those feelings.") Once the reasons are identified, discussions can begin about appropriate ways of expressing them. If feelings are expressed too vehemently, clients can alienate people who can help. Directed at the patient, they can cause hurt or confusion. The therapist can also discuss ways these clients can assert and take care of themselves, and advise them of ways to handle particular relationships. If it becomes clear that the anger is actually directed at the illness itself, this insight can serve to motivate the caregiver to work more actively with the patient against the illness (Jacobs, 2000). Given some form of expression, some issues causing anger are likely just to dissolve—and that might clear the way for the grief that lies underneath.

Grief

They are the silent griefs that cut the heartstrings."
John Ford, "The Broken Heart"

It is so natural to experience grief at all the losses cancer brings, as well as at the happy times that can no longer be. Although grief is natural, for many people it is the most painful of all emotions to endure. Even so, expressing their grief and loneliness is a productive way for family members to cope. When they do, they simply need acceptance and validation, not comfort. They do not need their sorrow fixed. Touching or trying to comfort people when they cry usually communicates only the request that they turn off their tears, not empathy. ("There, there, don't cry.") The best kind of help the therapist can give is to encourage their tears and their words:

- "You have every reason to grieve. You have lost so much."
- "Let the tears come. It's all right."
- "What are your tears saying? What are the words? You can talk and cry."
- "If all the pain and horror you are both going through are not worth some tears, then what is?"

Guilt

What is this self inside us, this silent observer,
Severe and speechless critic, who can terrorize us,
And urge us on to futile activity
And in the end, judge us still more severely . . . ?
T. S. Eliot, *The Elder Statesman*

Family members might feel guilty for what they see as all kinds of transgressions: for not having seen the illness coming, for not having spent more time with the patient before the diagnosis or now, for having taken the time to do something they enjoy, for feeling resentful, or for wishing that somehow the situation would just end. Very often the real underlying reason for their guilt is their belief that somehow they should be able to save the person they love, that they aren't saving him, and the fact remains that they themselves are well while the patient is ill.

While this kind of guilt is natural, unlike most emotions it is not healthy. Usually it is baseless, founded on false ideas. For these reasons, it needs to be challenged: questioned, explored, and reframed.

Reframing

We rarely, if ever, respond to events in our lives objectively. We react to the meaning we make of them. There are alternate ways to look at anything. Sometimes it isn't cancer itself but the meaning we attach to it that is so devastating. Reframing is shifting our perspective, changing the meaning. It can be an important part of therapy with people dealing with cancer, for it involves a different way of looking at their situation that makes it more bearable.

Emotions can be reframed, and when they are, they can become less overwhelming. The situation to which someone responds with intense grief or anxiety can be converted into a challenge or problem that can be managed one step at a time.

> Martha's husband, Ben, had a late-stage cancer. Conventional treatment had not helped, and Ben was in a clinical trial for an experimental drug. He was becoming increasingly debilitated by the aggressive treatment. His most recent tests showed that the cancer was growing. Martha said that since they learned about those test

results, "Ben has been upset, very sad, and scared. He's been crying a lot, and I hold him when he cries, but it's anguishing for me."

I explained that Ben's crying did not make his situation harder for him. On the contrary, it made it easier: less painful and less frightening. "When he cries and you hold him, you are helping him enormously. Even when he doesn't cry, you know he feels sad and afraid, no matter how optimistic he sounds. With his tears, he is simply letting out what he is feeling much of the time anyway. Crying is a wonderful release for him—emotionally and physically. By expressing his grief in this way, he doesn't have to use energy to hold it in or to pretend cheerfulness that he doesn't feel. Crying is exactly what he needs to do. When you hold him, you encourage him to cry. Maybe if you regard your holding him as one of the best kinds of help you can give him, and see him as doing something that is helping him emotionally, it might not be quite as anguishing for you."

The next time we spoke, she said that it was much easier for her to be close to Ben when he wept.

Fear and guilt based on distorted beliefs or on unrealistic, catastrophic thinking can also be changed. Statements like these, for example, should set off a loud mental alarm bell in the therapist:

- "The doctor didn't call back yet about the test results. That probably means that he has bad news."
- "A woman in my family support group has a son with the same kind of cancer as my husband. Now her son has a metastasis to his liver. I'm afraid that my husband will wind up the same way."
- "The oncologist said my daughter is responding well, but she's so sick from those treatments that I don't believe it. The cancer is probably spreading all through her body."
- "I know I should be strong, but sometimes I sure don't feel that way."

- "I've always had bad luck. Nothing ever goes my way."
- "If I had made him go to the doctor sooner, this wouldn't have happened."

Such baseless fears and guilt can be corrected, challenged, and reframed. Fears based on reality can be converted into a productive incentive to ask physicians questions about the illness or treatment about which the client has been concerned. Anger can also be redirected to asking for information from physicians, or requesting that they give more time and attention to the patient's needs.

Caregivers' view of their relationship with the patient can also be changed. Rather than seeing the patient as a helpless victim or themselves as overburdened martyrs, they can regard themselves and the patient as comrades fighting together for the patient's health and life.

Beliefs about the disease itself can also be reframed. Cancer can be seen not as invariably terminal, but as a manageable illness, whether it is temporary or chronic. A grim statistic can be seen not as an infallible forecast, but as an average drawn from clinical studies that does not apply to any individual. A dreaded next chemotherapy treatment can be seen as "one more treatment finished and one fewer to go." Any difficult medical treatments can be seen as life-saving gifts rather than painful torture. The patient's fatigue and nausea during chemotherapy need to be seen for what they are: side effects of the treatment, not symptoms of cancer.

Caregivers' beliefs about themselves can be changed. When the therapist reminds these clients of their strengths and discusses with them the many ways they can help the patient, their self-image can be changed. They can come to realize that there are some things (like saving someone from having cancer) that no one can do. Their view of themselves as helpless martyrs can be reframed so that they see themselves instead as active participants making a difference in their loved one's fight for life.

There is no one way, no one approach, to bring about the expression and, when necessary, the reframing of caregivers' emotions. The most effective way depends on the individual and the moment. Any psychotherapy approach, including Gestalt work (with the screaming and yelling it can entail), art therapy, or cognitive therapy, might help different clients at different times.

Whatever the therapy approach, a major aim of the work with many clients dealing with cancer is to convert their despair into hope. With these clients, instilling hope is the therapist's most important task. Hopelessness often is founded on misinformation and myths about cancer, ranging from the nonsensical to the downright dangerous. Identifying, correcting, and reframing them is one of the most important and helpful goals in therapy. Again, it is not groundless optimism that is wanted but rather an understanding of reality seen from the perspective of possibilities and hope.

CHAPTER 7

Ethical and Spiritual Aspects of the Work

Man lives in three dimensions: the somatic, the mental, and spiritual. The spiritual dimension cannot be ignored, for it is what makes us human.

Viktor Frankl, *The Doctor and the Soul* (1983, p. xvi)

In an attempt to be scientific, psychotherapy has claimed to be morally neutral and value-free—but in fact it is not. Every therapeutic dialogue presupposes and communicates values. It is almost impossible for therapists' moral, social, religious, and spiritual values and beliefs to play no part in their work. Therapists who believe that they do not make value judgments and that their approach is value-neutral are fooling themselves. Simply by nodding or not nodding they communicate their values. In other words, scientific objectivity in psychotherapy is not possible.

Besides being unrealistic, the idea of value-free psychotherapy has been recognized more and more to be based on outmoded and long-abandoned perspectives, and supplanted by perspectives involving moral values and spiritual ideas and beliefs. While ethical considerations and spiritual ideas have become more accepted as a part of psychotherapy, there is a wide variety of views about what this means and what it entails.

Mental health practitioners as a group have no clear and cogent concepts or standards with which to address moral or spiritual issues that arise in their work with clients. If and when such issues are discussed in therapy, it is important for both therapists and clients to recognize the values and beliefs they presuppose and make them explicit. This chapter discusses the place of ethical and spiritual values in psychotherapy with families dealing with cancer, and offers ethical and spiritual principles that can be included in a sound and meaningful way.

The Need for Ethical Considerations in Psychotherapy

Traditionally, psychology espoused the value of individual self-interest. Concepts of right and wrong, commitment, and obligation have had little or no place in psychotherapeutic dialogues. An individual's undesirable behavior was attributed to past influences of the family, community, environment, or culture. One family therapist, William Doherty (1999a), has pointed out that relationships have usually been discussed not in terms of responsibilities, but rather in terms of a self-interested benefits analysis for the client. Psychotherapists traditionally have promoted a morality of individual self-fulfillment. Commitments to others are seen as a means to the end of personal well-being, to be maintained as long as they work and discarded when they do not.

In recent years mental health practitioners have begun to recognize that the absence of moral values leads to the loss of self-respect, identity, and self-image. No one can grow when their responsibility is only to themselves. Growth has to do with the development and fulfillment of the possibilities of the self. One of these is the moral sense, a compassionate concern for others. The individual without such a commitment is not a fully developed human being. Neither is such an individual likely to find meaning and fulfillment in life. If we attribute someone's undesirable behavior to past influences over which he has no control, we leave no room for the possibilities of self-responsibility—which means no room for change and growth (Bolletino, 1998).

In working with family members caring for people with cancer, extremely difficult moral issues often arise. For example, family members might disagree with the patient's choice of medical treatments or with the patient's decision not to begin or continue treatment. Family members might find themselves having to make terrible decisions about whether they can maintain the quality of the patient's care in view of dwindling financial resources that affect others in the family. They might have to decide whether to keep a dying patient in the comfort and security of home when they themselves feel physically and emotionally drained and exhausted by ongoing efforts to provide care. Such situations lead them to ask themselves, "What is the right thing to do?"

Even though value-free therapy is not possible, psychotherapists cannot make moral decisions for their clients. It is certainly not our place to make moral pronouncements and certainly not our role to impose our own values and beliefs on clients. It is not our place even to give moral advice any more than it is to judge or give advice about clients' life choices. Nevertheless, for us to help these clients, we need to deal somehow with moral issues. The question is how.

The Need for Spiritual Considerations in Psychotherapy

In recent years our culture has been permeated with what has been called the New Spirituality, challenging psychotherapists to address the spiritual concerns of their clients. This spiritual explosion differs in significant ways from the kinds of spirituality expressed historically in major spiritual traditions (Bolletino, 2001).

The New Spirituality involves a multitude of diverse beliefs and practices, many of them free-floating fragments of teachings from other times and places, now no longer connected to theoretical or traditional contexts, or to experience. The situation is confusing.

Some clients in therapy are influenced by this cultural phenomenon. For that reason it is useful to ask whether therapists ought to take seriously what we hear from them about spirituality, and what we read and hear about it in the mass media as well as in some professional journals, workshops, and conferences. Without critical questioning, we might easily conclude that to become truly spiritual, what we all need to do, among other things, is to use crystals; meditate; trust our intuition; love and forgive everyone; communicate with the dead, with angels, or with channeled spirits; think only positive thoughts; respect the planet; read inspirational literature; attend spiritual lectures and workshops; maintain tranquility; engage in Western religious practices as well as those of Native American, Asian, and Middle Eastern religions; perform kind acts for people and animals; eat organic food; visualize; pray; breathe mindfully; consult the *I Ching*, astrologers, psychics, past-life therapists, energy workers, feng shui specialists, healers, gurus, or psychics; and finally, plan for a transcendent death and a happy reunion with our loved ones. These considerations bring to mind a line from Gilbert and Sullivan's *The Mikado*: "There's the idiot who praises with enthusiastic tone every century but this and every country but his own" (Bolletino, 2001). Theodore Rosak's description of the New Age movement of the 1960s still applies today: "We begin to resemble nothing as much as the cultic hothouse . . . [in ancient Greece], where every manner of mystery and fakery, ritual and rite intermingled with marvelous indiscrimination" (1969/1995, p. 78).

Spirituality is often regarded today as being free from the shackles of reason and intellect. Some people view it as anti-intellectual and anti-scientific, and associate it with the occult, magic, mysticism, or beings from outer space. Some regard it as something separate from the body, while others regard the path to it as being of or through the body. Sometimes spirituality is equated with religion, and sometimes it is not. When it comes to health, it is often assumed that any belief or practice described and regarded as spiritual is ipso facto healing. Many people seeking a cure for specific problems (including cancer) consult practitioners they regard as spiritual.

The New Spirituality is reflected in professional psychology as well as our popular culture. For at least three decades, many psychologists and psychiatrists have been attracted to the teachings of Zen and Tibetan Buddhism, Sufism, various forms of Hinduism, the practices of early monastic and Eastern Christianity, and certain surviving remnants of mystical Judaism—Kabbalah and Hasidism. They have engaged in much activity and theorizing about these teachings. The humanistic and existentialist schools of psychology have directed their focus to transpersonal psychology, studying, for example, nonordinary states of consciousness, mind-expanding substances, yoga, and peak experiences. In some part of the United States mental health clinics openly tie their treatment to fundamentalist Christianity, while many schools of therapy have developed around mystical New Age beliefs (Watters & Ofshe, 1999).

Beyond a lack of agreement about what spirituality is, there is also no consensus concerning standards for judging ideas about spirituality. People use different criteria for determining whether a statement in this area has meaning, whether a line of reasoning has validity or a theory has coherence. Unfortunately, many people believe that all knowledge is subjective, so that any belief about spirituality is regarded to be as true as any other, and any theory as sound as any other. Because spirituality is often regarded as separate from reason and therefore free of its constraints, many disparate notions, no matter how far removed from experience, are often accepted without question and grafted somehow onto a body of accepted beliefs.

In both the professional and popular literature, spirituality is sometimes conceived as being unconnected to the ethical realm of interpersonal responsibility. At its worst, the literature treats the individual as an unencumbered spiritual being, free to grow and explore with little attention to obligation and concern for others. Some writers assume that spiritual enlightenment automatically leads to morally sensitive behavior, even though that is not necessarily the case (Doherty, 1999b).

Many thoughtful observers have remarked on the emptiness, and on the self-satisfying, even narcissistic, ideas and practices of current spirituality. The philosopher Jacob Needleman (1977) wrote that we use concepts that are naive and hollow, and adopt the terminology, the props and the practices without changing anything essential in our inner lives. He also observed that unlike every serious spiritual movement in history that has included an ethical element, a deep conviction of concern and help for others, the New Spirituality has an inner focus. Although it preaches unconditional love, it rarely advocates the responsibility to demonstrate this with the people around us. Instead, it often seems to be about self-absorption and about ways to feel good, with no meaning beyond that. In Western cultures, real spiritual development calls for action (Needleman, 1977).

Thomas Moore, a former Catholic monk and the author of *Care of the Soul,* wrote,

> We in America are losing our deep spirituality even as many celebrate an apparent renaissance of the transcendent kind. I am not so enthusiastic about the supposed renaissance because I see much narcissism in it . . . in the project of making a superior self. (1998, p. 41)

In view of all this, another line from Gilbert and Sullivan, this one from *Patience,* comes to mind: "The meaning doesn't matter if it's only idle chatter of a transcendental kind."

But it isn't all only idle chatter. The New Spirituality arose in response to universal needs for meaning and purpose that are not being adequately filled in our society today. They are universal in that we know of no culture or period in history in which there was not evidence of these needs. In every culture we know of, people have perceived that there is a dimension of human beings that cannot be described or accounted for in psychological, intellectual, or physical terms alone. That "something else" can best be called our spiritual aspect.

The New Spirituality, however, offers no serious or profound understanding for making inner change. All the great spiritual traditions of the world involve ideas that cannot be grasped, much less lived, without extraordinary commitment and intelligence, as well as prolonged help from others who have gone through the necessary stages of the path themselves (Needleman, 1997). Much of the New Spirituality requires no commitment of disciplined study, training, and practice.

Further, unlike every major spiritual movement in history, which includes a deep commitment to concern and help for others, the New Spirituality has no underlying ethical component. It is a kind of street bazaar with vendors hawking their wares while customers fill shopping bags with jumbles of ideas, objects, rituals, and practices.

In its popular forms, the New Spirituality has had deleterious effects on some clients, for it has help to seed many of them with nonsensical ideas. As discussed in an earlier chapter, some of these ideas are psychologically toxic. For example, one is that we create our reality, which means we also create our own misfortunes—including cancer. This has led many cancer patients and their families to feelings of helplessness, guilt, and inadequacy when they cannot succeed in creating their own cure. Another is that to be truly spiritual, we must banish negative emotions and be serene at all times. This, too, arouses guilt in clients who somehow cannot seem to manage to maintain serenity in the face of a life-threatening illness.

It is impossible to believe that these ideas are spiritual, that they arise out of a sense of spirituality, or even that they are exclusive to people who view themselves as spiritual. Rather, they are baseless pseudo-metaphysical presumptions that have proliferated as the result of the prevalence of pop spirituality. Mental health professionals, who are likely to hear them from clients dealing with cancer in their lives, are well advised to recognize their implications and effects on those clients.

The New Spirituality also has had deleterious effects on the practice of therapy and psychology. First, as it has washed over American culture, it has encouraged people to believe that spirituality is somehow a quick and easy fix for psychological and even physical problems. (This has actually prevented some cancer patients from seeking medical treatments.) The other unfortunate effect is that people have embraced many free-floating ideas of the New Spirituality that are at best irrelevant to their psychological growth. Equally unfortunate is that some therapists have been encouraged to include in their practices so-called spiritual words, ideas, and perspectives that have no more substance than the marketplace array of the New Spirituality.

To put it bluntly, clients influenced by popular thought and legitimately yearning for something more come to therapy with absurd notions about spirituality (for examples see Chapter 4). Some therapists they encounter have equally nonsensical ideas. To say the least, this impedes progress in therapy.

Of course if psychology had sound, meaningful, and rooted concepts of spirituality, the effect of the New Spirituality would be minimal, even if clients did arrive for therapy with silly ideas. But professional psychology traditionally has ignored, discounted, or even pathologized clients' statements about their spiritual or religious experiences and beliefs. For the most part, spirituality itself has been viewed as a foolish and irrelevant notion, despite the efforts over the past 50 years of a number of psychiatrists, psychologists, and therapists to develop fruitful theories attempting to integrate spirituality into psychotherapy. They include William James, Carl Jung, Robert Assagioli, Abraham Maslow, Gordon Allport, Stanislov Graf, and Viktor Frankl. (To describe and acknowledge their individual contributions, another book would be needed.)

In recent years we have learned too much about the positive effects of spiritual and religious beliefs to disregard them, particularly for clients dealing with life-threatening illnesses. Such beliefs influence the ways we live, the ways we act toward others, and the ways we respond to good fortune, adversity, and tragedy. When we are trying to cope with illness, pain, and suffering, our beliefs influence our reactions to the illness and our expectations about its future course.

As a result of all this, mental health professionals face a critical challenge. Many people who come to psychotherapy, certainly including those dealing with cancer, are seeking help in finding purpose and meaning in their lives. They are seeking ways to deal with the situation they face and to make sense of it. They are seeking ways to touch something deep inside them that has been untouched. Many come seeking to discover what is of value for themselves, or to try to resolve difficult practical, emotional, or moral conflicts. They are seeking to transcend who they are now.

The New Spirituality has pushed mental health professionals to open themselves more broadly than ever before to the spiritual concerns of both their clients and themselves. But given the nonspiritual tradition of their respective professions, therapists as a group have no clear, cogent standards by which to acknowledge and meet those concerns or to allow clients their own integrity in the course of therapy.

What might such standards be? The question is, how can spirituality be included in the practice of psychotherapy in a clear, disciplined, and meaningful way? Psychotherapy is a practical field. If we believe that human beings have a spiritual dimension they need to express in order to grow and be "fully" human, we must be very clear about what this means and what it entails. Regardless of the school of therapy we represent, we must be clear about where we are going.

The Relationship of Spirituality and Religion

The use of the word *spirituality* here is not intended to imply a necessarily religious connotation. Spirituality and religion are not the same thing. Spirituality is the basis or core of religion; religion is the systemization or codification of spirituality. Sometimes when spirituality is codified, it is lost. While spirituality sometimes takes the form of a religious commitment, it can, and often does, exist without religion. While there are great varieties of religions, spirituality is common to all human beings. In whatever ways spirituality is conceptualized, it is clear that, as Viktor Frankl said, it is "the capacity we possess that is uniquely human."

The Fundamental Ethical Principle for Psychotherapy

Chapter 3 presented principles for an effective approach for people dealing with cancer. They serve as axioms or presuppositions that can guide the work, defining the way we interact with the people who come to us as clients. They are also moral principles, defining the basis of professional practice.

The fundamental principle is that each client needs to be seen and treated as a unique individual. This axiom not only underlies effective therapy, but is also its most fundamental ethical principle. Let us examine just what it means and what it entails, since it has a number of implications.

The first implication is that each client needs to be seen and treated as a whole person. In many ways, all of us human beings are similar. In at least as many ways, each of us is different. We can know a client only if we see her in her totality. This cannot happen if we see only some of her aspects, or if we summarize her by reducing her to an example of some abstract classification, such as a *DSM* category or the category of family caregivers. Only if the therapist recognizes and responds to the client's total being can that client be helped.

People often see only what they expect to see, and fail to see what they don't expect. When, as therapists, we look at someone through a diagnostic lens, we see only what is wrong and disregard almost everything else. Even if a client fully fits a diagnosis, there is much else about the person we might be ignoring or about which we are unaware. As we get to know her, we see how that individual is different from others, including others in the same diagnostic category to which she has been assigned. The better we come to know the person and to recognize her complexity and uniqueness, the more any category with which she has been identified fades. Generally speaking, the more a client appears to us to fit into a diagnosis, the less we know about the person because we have lost sight of that individual. Seeing someone clearly involves recognizing all her complex aspects as a total person.

In short, the therapist needs to encounter each client as a whole, unique individual and build a relationship from that.

Second, to see and treat the client as a total human being involves recognizing and respecting the person's autonomy, the ability to make choices and bring about change.

Viewing the person as a product of heredity, past influences, or environment, for example, or as a pawn of instinctual drives and reactions is inconsistent with seeing him as a total, autonomous human being. All of us are all influenced and shaped by our past, but unless we assume that we are free to shape our future and are capable of doing so, psychotherapy is pointless.

Third, to see and treat each client as a total, autonomous individual, the therapist must understand that clients are the leading world authorities on themselves. The therapist cannot presume to know more about a client than the client does. While the therapist might be an expert on psychotherapy, clients are the only experts on who they are and what they need.

Fourth, because each person is like no other, no psychological theory can apply to everyone, and no prefabricated technique can be equally effective for everyone. In the past, most therapists believed that there was one right way of doing therapy: the way their mentor or school had taught them. They usually assumed that if they learned that method well enough, they would cure their clients. No one seemed to notice that different therapists, using different methods, were achieving comparable results (LeShan, 1996).

In view of all this, therapy is best when it can be spontaneous, flowing from a unique encounter with the client from moment to moment. Carl Jung wrote:

It is enough to drive one to despair that in practical psychology there are no universally valid recipes and rules. There are only individual cases with the most heterogeneous needs and demands—so heterogeneous that we can virtually never know in advance what course a given case will take, for which reason it is better for the doctor to abandon all preconceived opinions. (1978, p. 81)

He also wrote:

Experience has taught me to keep away from therapeutic methods as much from diagnoses. The enormous variations among individuals . . . [have] set before me the ideal of approaching each case with a minimum of prior assumptions. The ideal would naturally be to have no assumption at all. But this is impossible. (1978, p. 81)

The therapist Florence Miale said that any of the therapist's responses that come from technique instead of human feelings are antitherapeutic. Echoing the call for spontaneity, the psychiatrist Irving Yalom pointed out that standardized protocols, procedures, and diagnostic formulations merely obstruct the possibility of knowing the client as deeply as possible. He suggested that therapists would do well to "create a new therapy for each client" that happens in an unpremeditated response to each moment (Yalom, 2003, p. 34)

Fifth, the only way that therapists can come to understand and respond to clients as total, unique individuals is to be genuinely and emotionally involved. It is not possible to tune into what another person feels without allowing ourselves to be emotionally open. Involvement has nothing to do with therapeutic techniques or methods and does not conflict with seeing another person clearly. The therapist must really care about the patient, and the patient's becoming. Part of this caring is faith in the patient's ability to change and grow in whatever ways he or she needs to.

Therapists learn to distance themselves emotionally and adopt a neutral, so-called "objective" viewpoint not simply because objectivity is the viewpoint of science. Their emotional distancing serves to separate and protect them from their own feelings of helplessness and grief in the face of emotional suffering, sorrow, death, and loss. It is a natural reaction for anyone in certain circumstances to erect a protective shield of detachment, usually without being aware that they do so. However, maintaining an objective stance is not conductive to the client's growth—and the aim of therapy is to promote that growth. In other words, because the therapist's detachment is contrary to the aim of therapy, it is unethical. Effective therapy, particularly with clients in crisis, depends on large part on the humanness of the therapist. The therapist must be deeply concerned about the person. People dealing with cancer need understanding and support. A therapist who is impersonal and uninvolved does not offer this. Rather than an objective viewpoint, what is needed might be called *disciplined subjectivity*.

As therapist and client come to know each other better, they are less and less in their respective roles. They come to know each other's depths and to feel a special closeness and trust born from what they have shared of themselves. However, although their relationship is characterized by a shared purpose, it is not one of equality and mutuality. No matter how close they feel, it is always the therapist, not the client, who is the caregiver. It is always the therapist, not the client, who is alert to the other's needs, and who gives encouragement, reassurance, hope, and comfort. While the client comes to know the therapist as a human being, the therapist does not express many of the feelings and needs that the work engenders. Further, during any session, there is a total commitment on the therapist's part to the client's growth and becoming. There should be no such commitment on the part of the client.

It is apparent that clients can grow and progress with therapists who are emotionally open and caring. Perhaps it is not as apparent that therapists benefit as well. Although they risk emotional distress by working with people dealing with a life-threatening illness, experienced practitioners find that the more open they are, the greater their rewards. They learn that allowing themselves to be open does not damage them, and it makes their work more rewarding, meaningful, and fulfilling. They learn that their caring teaches their clients to care about themselves, and so provides the ground for further positive development.

Moral Issues in the Therapeutic Dialogue

A therapist cannot know a client without knowing and understanding the person's beliefs and values. Again, it is not the therapist's place to make moral pronouncements, to dictate, or even to offer moral prescriptions or advice. Psychotherapists are not gurus, judges, or arbiters in moral or spiritual matters, and it is surely unethical for them to impose their own values.

What they can do is point out the moral considerations involved in some of the decisions their clients make. They can discuss with clients what each regards as the fair, right, honest, or responsible course of action in a given situation. The therapist can encourage clients' moral sense by helping them to recognize, clarify, and apply their own moral values.

This does not mean that the therapist needs to adopt a moral relativism by accepting all the client's values as equally good. It is the therapist's responsibility to challenge destructive, nihilist, or deterministic values and ideas, and to raise questions about the ramifications of the clients' actions for others as well as for themselves.

By strengthening clients' moral sense, the therapist conveys respect for them as moral agents and provides a framework in which they can change and grow in terms of their own values. The therapist's respect for the moral agency of the client is the safeguard protecting discussions about moral values from becoming prescriptive and coercive (Doherty, 1999b). By strengthening clients' moral sense, the therapist also strengthens their sense of self, including ethical empowerment and self-respect.

Family caregivers often tend to be concerned about helping the cancer patient while ignoring or neglecting their own needs. Some tend to regard the patient as far more important than themselves and to make sacrificial decisions. However, self-respect and respect for others are inextricably intertwined. The psychiatrist Frieda Fromm-Reichmann (1960) pointed out that one can respect others only to the extent that one respects oneself. In other words, there is no contradiction between self-fulfillment and moral responsibility to others. The question in each situation is how best to respect and value everyone involved.

Moral Characteristics of the Therapist

The ability to introduce moral consideration in psychotherapy ultimately rests on the moral character of the therapist.

Honesty is viewed by some therapists as a means of establishing trust rather than as a moral obligation. Caring, the unqualified concern for the client's welfare, is often viewed as a means of establishing and maintaining a therapeutic bond rather than a moral characteristic. Courage is rarely recognized as a necessary moral quality (Doherty, 1999b).

Yet people who come to therapy have a right to hear from us what is true. Besides honesty, caring is the heart of the therapeutic process. Caring does not conflict with our ability to see our clients clearly. It entails deep concern about the client and the client's becoming. It also entails faith in the client's ability to grow in whatever ways he or she needs. (Freud, asked why psychoanalysis cures the patient, replied that it is because there is a moment in which the therapist loves the patient, and the patient knows it and is cured.)

Courage is also required. To work with people involved with cancer, we sometimes need nerves of steel to discuss what we sometimes would rather not talk about, and to confront ourselves, our feelings, and our mistakes (Doherty, 1999a). We need courage to put aside our fears in examining issues of life and death.

We also need humility. We must be humble enough, as the psychiatrist Elisabeth Kübler-Ross said, to know that we, too, need healing: "If [psychotherapists] are too arrogant to acknowledge this, the whole interaction is contaminated" (1989, p. 128). The therapist Hugh Prather made the same point: "The mind that sees itself as whole and another as sick unquestionably requires healing" (1989, p. 16). Anyone working as a psychotherapist requires many years of therapy. To believe otherwise is a colossal form of arrogance. It was Jung who pointed out that a therapist can help clients only as far as the therapist himself has gone, and "not a step further" (1978, p. 90). When a client gets stuck, it is usually at the point where the therapist could make no further progress herself. Without having had years of personal therapy, the therapist is saying in effect, "Do as I say, not as I do." Besides years of therapy, every therapist, no matter how experienced, also needs a supervisor to remain open to another point of view. As Jung put it, "Even the pope has a confessor" (1965, p. 134).

The psychiatrist Viktor Frankl wrote that the meaning of our work as psychotherapists is what we bring to it as human beings (1995). Jung made the same point when he said that everything depends on the therapist and little or nothing on the method (1989).

The Primacy of the Person

It is the thesis here that one fundamental ethical principle governs the practice of psychotherapy. It is the foundation from which all other ethical principles and all rules of professional conduct are derived, and it serves as the criterion for all professional decisions and actions: The therapist is to regard each client with unconditional, unremitting concern and respect as a unique human being with intrinsic worth and the ability to structure his own life. Every code of professional conduct rests on this principle.

There are no clear-cut rules for applying this principle in every situation. What is critical is that the practitioner's perceptions, attitudes, deliberations, and decisions are shaped by this moral law. It will be helpful here to consider some implications for professional practice and examples of ways in which the principle can be violated.

First, psychotherapists normally expect to set regularly scheduled office appointments, lasting 45, 50, or 60 minutes, for which clients pay an agreed-upon fee. There are policies about late arrivals, cancellations, and missed sessions. Along with boundaries concerning place, time, regularity, and payment, we also set emotional boundaries. As professionals, self-disclosure and expression of our emotional responses are carefully considered. We are expected to reveal our feelings or facts about ourselves rarely and judiciously.

These policies and expectations can become unrealistic and at times counterproductive with clients dealing with cancer in the family. Clients might be needed to care for the patient and have to cancel or change appointments. They might be able to schedule sessions only infrequently or irregularly, or only for irregular times or durations. Because of high medical expenses in their families, or inadequate or canceled insurance, they might be unable to pay the usual fee.

Clearly it is a basic right of any professional to set and consistently maintain policies and boundaries that apply to all clients. On the other hand, a refusal to change policies can be regarded as abandonment when a client is unable to comply with them. Practitioners' refusal or inability to extend their emotional boundaries can also be experienced by these clients as a kind of abandonment. If practitioners maintain a "professional" emotional detachment, or remain uninvolved, cold, distant, joyless, or out of touch with themselves, the client is alone.

Second, in view of the primacy principle that each person is to be seen and treated as total, unique person, it is unethical (as well as counterproductive for the therapy) to regard and treat the client in terms of a diagnosis or any abstract category.

Third, arrogance on the part of the therapist is antithetical to the primacy principle as well as a violation of the client. Arrogance can take many forms. One form is the assumption that we know what is best for our clients, or that we can understand them better than they know or understand themselves. The reality is that every individual knows more about herself than anyone else possibly can. To assume otherwise is to disrespect the person.

Another form of arrogance is the presumption that we may make decisions for the client or impose them on the client. Even the assumption that we can give meaningful advice to the client can deny the person as being a capable and responsible agent.

Still another form of arrogance is the attempt to impose any of our own personal religious or spiritual beliefs. (If the therapist incorporates in her work any particular religious viewpoint or any spiritual practices, this should be made clear to prospective clients in advance. If not, the therapist is being dishonest.) Particularly with clients whose family member is seriously or even terminally ill, and who are deeply vulnerable, for a practitioner even to suggest a possible religious viewpoint or concept is inappropriate and intrusive.

Psychotherapists often feel that when the patient is seriously ill, the family members ought to be talking about dying or about spiritual matters, and that the person's failure to do so is denial. The reality is that in these situations, the need to talk about dying is often the practitioner's, not the client's. Whatever the client does or does not talk about is her choice. Those practitioners who respect their client will simply be present, allowing the client to decide what to discuss. To impose any subject matter or belief is a violation and an abuse of power. For example, a client whose family member is terminally ill might ask the therapist, "Do you believe there is life after death?" The only moral answer to this is, "What is that you believe? That's all that's important."

Another form of arrogance is the assumption that the kind of therapy we offer is right for everyone. This assumption denies the uniqueness of each individual client. A variation of this assumption is that no advanced specialized training or supervision is needed to work with anyone seeking therapy. A notable example is that some therapists with little or no training or experience with clients dealing with life-threatening illnesses do not hesitate to accept cancer patients or their family members as new clients, apparently believing that they are fully qualified to work with them.

Applying the fundamental principle of primacy involves recognizing that it is always the client, not the therapist, who is the one to determine what is meaningful. Rather than imposing values and meaning by any kind of manipulation or coercion—be it by suggestion, insinuation, or persuasion—the therapist can help make it possible for clients to make decisions that help to develop and strengthen their sense of responsibility and self-empowerment. The attitude that is wanted is always unconditional respect. This means faith in each client's ability to create a meaningful life that is uniquely his, and to express his ethical and spiritual dimension in his own individual way.

What therapists can provide is their conviction that there are values and meanings in life that are available to everyone. In Viktor Frankl's words, "Life retains its meaning under any conditions. It remains meaningful literally up to the last moment, up to the last breath" (1985, p. 121).

The principle of the primacy of the person underlies all other ethical principles and serves as a criterion for assessing the ethical validity of professional attitudes, decisions, and actions. Ethical behavior cannot be legislated. However, there is more and more evidence that seeing and treating a client as something less than a whole, unique, autonomous person is antitherapeutic. Because it is psychologically harmful, it is unethical.

Spirituality in Psychotherapy

How can spirituality be conceived so that it can be included in a relevant and meaningful way in professional practice? The primary aim of any kind of psychotherapy is the growth and health of the individual as an integrated whole. Any concept of spirituality must be consistent with that aim.

To have relevant meaning, a concept of spirituality has to involve far more than just believing something, talking about something, reading or thinking about something, or even doing something. It needs to be an attitude, a consistent perspective, a way of looking at the world that is expressed in the way we live and the way we experience our lives.

A very general concept of spirituality has been expressed historically in the principle that life is sacred. Albert Einstein called this "the supreme value to which all values are subordinate" (1982). Albert Schweitzer called it "the reverence for life," which he described as "the principle in which affirmation of the world and ethics are joined together" (1998). This principle has been described not simply as an abstract idea, but as a perception that comes from experience and reflection.

For psychotherapy, the most significant part of this principle is that the people who entrust themselves to our care are to be regarded as sacred. This means that each person is inviolate. The recognition of the sanctity and inviolability of human beings becomes a living axiom, informing our attitudes, decisions, and actions as psychotherapists.

It is the thesis here that spirituality in psychotherapy is about the sacredness of each person. There is an intrinsic preciousness in human beings that is not present in insentient matter. This concept of spirituality is at least as old as the Old Testament, in which it is written that human beings were created in the image of the Divine. There are no rules or correct methods for applying this fundamental spiritual axiom. The practitioner's constant awareness of the client's sacredness is what brings spirituality into the psychotherapy office. With this view, that room becomes holy ground. When we have this awareness, it is as if each client we are with speaks to us the words of the poet William Butler Yeats: "I have spread my dreams under your feet. Tread softly because you tread on my dreams."

Summary and Conclusion

Applied to psychotherapy, the principle of the primacy of the person underlies all other ethical principles and serves as a criterion for assessing the ethical validity of professional decisions and actions. Ethical behavior cannot be legislated. However, there is more and more evidence that seeing and treating a client as something less than as a whole, unique, autonomous person is antitherapeutic. It is psychologically harmful and therefore unethical. As an ethical and spiritual concept, the principle of primacy advances the most basic aim of psychotherapy: the growth of the individual as a whole person.

The therapist's attitudes and behavior are critical because the therapist is a model for the client. To paraphrase Lawrence LeShan (1996), when the therapist listens to the client, the client learns to listen to himself. When the therapist cares about the client, the client learns to care about herself. When the therapist has hopes for the client, the client learns to have hopes for himself. When the therapist trusts and respects the client, the client comes to trust and respect herself. And when the therapist loves the client by being responsible to her and committed to her welfare, the client learns to be committed and responsible to others as well as herself. When the therapist sees the client as sacred and inviolable, the client learns to see himself and other human beings in this way.

When I was a young child, there was a moment in which I saw living things in a different way than I had ever seen them before. I was watching a butterfly fluttering around the leaves of a tree. Until then I had taken the natural world for granted, assuming that it was mine to do with what I liked. At that moment, though, for the first time I became aware that the butterfly and the tree were alive, and I knew I did not understand why or how this was so. Both the tree and the butterfly had become amazing mysteries. For the first time I knew with certainty that because they were alive I must not interfere with them or harm them. Looking back at that experience, I can say that it was the first time I saw life as holy and inviolable.

Now, as a therapist, I have the same feeling when I am invited into a client's innermost being, into the miracle of the person's living soul. At those times, it is not possible to be unaware of the person's spiritual dimension or of my own.

Carl Jung had a sign above his office door, reminding his patients and himself that their work together was spiritual as well as psychological: "Whether or not he is called, the God will be present." ("Vocatus atque non vocatus, Deus aderit.")

For both professionals and clients a similar perspective is needed.

PART II

HELPING THE FAMILY CAREGIVER HELP THE PATIENT

CHAPTER 8

The Experiential World of the Person With Cancer

What goes through your mind when you're lying, full of nuclear dye, under a huge machine that scans all your bones for evidence of treason? There's a horror-movie appeal to the machine. Beneath it you become the Frankenstein monster exposed to the electric storm. How do you appear to yourself when you sit with bare shins and no underwear beneath a scanty cotton gown in a hospital waiting room? Nobody, not even a lover, waits as intensely as a critically ill patient.

Anatole Broyard, *Intoxicated by My Illness* (1992, p. 22)

The emotional responses to having cancer are at least as painful as the illness itself. People who become patients are thrust into an alien world where even their bodies are unfamiliar. (One patient described it as being abducted to a strange land where the terrain, customs and language are unknown; Broyard, 1992). For those who have never been on the receiving end of a cancer diagnosis and who care for someone with that illness, the intense and changing emotions of the patient can be easily misunderstood or minimized. Family and professional caregivers, who are all dealing with their own emotional reactions to the person's diagnosis, try to understand what the patient is experiencing so that they can be as supportive as possible. However, we can never underestimate the distance between being in physical and emotional pain and trying to empathize with it.

Besides not always understanding the patient's emotions, family members sometimes misinterpret or resent them, or believe that some of those responses (the so-called negative emotions) will make the patient sicker. Often they simply do not know how to react, what to do, what to say, or how to express what they want to say. Sometimes patients themselves don't know what they feel because their feelings are so complex and so strong. Too often they, like their family members, believe that they should not be having the feelings that they do, and that there must be something psychologically wrong with them. Far too often health care practitioners also mistake these natural reactions for psychological problems.

Having cancer, Lawrence LeShan wrote, is like waking each morning to a nightmare—not a bad dream, but a nightmare, with a nightmare's special psychologically weakening and physically exhausting effects. A nightmare has three characteristics. First, terrible things are happening and worse are threatened. Second, we feel helpless, impotent while other people or outside forces are in control. Third, there is no time limit, no end in sight. Being trapped in the nightmare of cancer weakens the coherence of the person's sense of self (LeShan, 1994).

"What is the hardest thing about having cancer?" I asked Magda, a 60-year-old woman with ovarian cancer, shortly after our first session began. Without needing to think for even a moment, she answered unhesitatingly: "It's always there."

Cancer is thus usually an overwhelming psychological trauma. The main characteristic of this kind of trauma is frequently terror. Traumatic events are those that produce intense fear, helplessness, loss of control, and the threat of annihilation. While every individual is different, Phil's story will illustrate a broad spectrum of emotions that is not at all unusual.

Phil felt as if every part of his life was becoming infected, and that he was spreading the infection to everyone around him. Often he was impatient and irritable with the people he cared about most even as he realized they were trying to help him. He disliked himself when he behaved this way but didn't know how to stop. Neither could he stop himself when he needed to make his wife, Jenny, understand how terrible he felt, and then he disliked himself even more for causing her this distress.

Often on edge, he drove too fast, shouting and shaking his fist at drivers who impeded him. Jenny was afraid to get in the car with him. It wasn't just bad drivers who enraged him. Most of all it was the politicians in Washington and, for that matter, anyone else in the world who seemed blind to injustice.

He felt that his illness caused him to become a burden to Jenny and their teenage son Jon, so he tried hard to put in as many work hours as he could, handle some household chores, and tell Jenny often how much he appreciated her help and patience. Sometimes, though, after chemotherapy treatments, he was so tired that everything was too much. At those times, when it seemed that it was the cancer and not he who was in charge, he became despondent. Two years earlier, not long after he was first diagnosed, when life seemed to have become only cancer and treatments with no way out, he had come close to trying to kill himself. At that time he spoke to no one, certainly not to Jenny, about how he felt. His plan was to jump in front of a railroad train—but then he realized that he was too frightened to do it and didn't really want to.

A year later tests showed that the cancer had spread. It was shortly after he recovered from surgery and began chemotherapy again that he came to see me. With two degrees in electrical engineering, Phil was a freelance writer for several technical journals. (His articles were highly technical. At my request he once sent me a copy of one. On it he had written, "Read this whenever you have trouble sleeping.") When we began working together, on most days he was still going to the small office he had rented for at least a few hours, writing and marketing his articles, and coming home to his supportive family. Nevertheless he sometimes felt lost, as if, like a character in Solzhenitsyn's novel *The Cancer Ward*, the familiar ordered life he had known was "on the other side of his tumor." Now after nearly 2 years of oppressive and almost continuous illness and treatments, at times he could easily swing between anger, sadness, fear, despair, and depression, as well as enthusiasm, humor, and love.

As Phil was learning, many of the reactions evoked by a cancer diagnosis are neither cheerful nor pleasant.

Shock, Disbelief, Denial, and Vulnerability

Even though we might have suspected the diagnosis of cancer, when we hear it we are totally unprepared. We feel shock coupled with psychological and physiological pain. As the shock lessens, we feel utter disbelief, then terror and bewilderment. We are unable to think clearly. Like the experience of the people who love and care for us, nothing seems real, nothing seems immediate. We are disoriented, as if we are living in a dream. Everything is at a distance as if we are surrounded by a protective covering that numbs us. We are protecting ourselves against our terrifying and paralyzing thought that we are helpless against a mysterious, deadly enemy that has invaded our body and can kill us. ("This can't be happening," "The diagnosis is wrong," "I'm really not sick at all," "Not me. I've always taken good care of myself," "No, it can't be true. I feel perfectly healthy.") Our denial helps us to function and stay calm.

Usually, as things settle down—often when a course of treatment is decided on and begun and we find that we can handle it, our shock eases. However, like all our other emotions, denial can come and go.

For example, months after his surgery and during his chemotherapy treatment, Ray, another cancer patient, said, "On the whole, I'm feeling all right. Whenever the doctor says anything, I have the feeling he isn't talking to me."

Denial is a survival mechanism, allowing us to filter in reality little by little as we are ready to deal with it. As with caregivers, however, if denial persists, it can prevent the patient from taking appropriate action when action is called for. This might take the form of refusing to go for medical treatment on the ground that the cancer will just go away, perhaps if the patient starts a special diet, or meditates, or just visualizes it gone. When denial persists in this way, some patients ignore the obvious changes in their bodies while their cancer grows.

The initial shock might not be the only one. One patient described his entire experience with cancer as "a series of shocks."

Anxiety, Fear, and Terror

Present dangers are less than horrible imaginings.
William Shakespeare, *Macbeth* (I, iii, 34)

While cancer can erode the body, fear can erode the soul.

Just beneath the detachment, under the need to reject what is happening—and not always far under—are extreme anxiety, fear, and terror. There are no promises, no guarantee of a cure. We lose our sense of safety and our strong sense of self, and feel childlike in our vulnerability. We are terrified that we will die, or at least that we will never again live normally. We feel vulnerable as never before. We're terrified that we will be in unbearable pain; that our bodies won't work, that the treatment will fail, and that no one can help. At times our apprehension has no limits: We don't know what will happen; we fear all that we imagine can possibly happen; and our very existence feels threatened. These fears—of death, endless sickness, pain, helplessness, and the unknown—often stay with us unremittingly, like a heavy, silent, gray fog that never lifts, clouding our every experience.

Many fears are not unrealistic. We are afraid of losing strength and energy, feeling sick and weak, and becoming dependent. We are afraid of making treatment decisions we cannot know how to make, when all of our choices might be the wrong ones. We are afraid of intrusive treatments, and of encounters with intimidating, impersonal technology. We are afraid of being assaulted, damaged, and disfigured.

If we undergo surgery, chemotherapy, or radiation, we are terrified of the treatments themselves as well as their effects. Any of these treatments can produce physical changes that can devastate our lives. It is easy to forget why we are submitting to them. We dread every doctor's appointment, every treatment, every test, and every test result. Every ache, every twinge, every cough can become sinister. We are afraid the cancer will spread. We are afraid of losing more control of our bodies and our lives, and of becoming more dependent on others. We are apprehensive about the emotional and financial burdens our illness places on us and our families, and about its effects on every aspect of our lives.

Sometimes we are anxious, even panicked, without knowing exactly why. Fear is always one step behind us, drawing closer when we do not give it voice. We are constantly aware that we might not go on living. T. S. Eliot's J. Alfred Prufrock spoke for us when he said, "I have seen the eternal footman hold my coat, and snicker, and in short, I was afraid." Whether it is in the foreground or recedes for a while into the background, fear stalks us relentlessly even when we sleep, and we feel it in every part of our ourselves.

We might also feel horror that our body has been attacked, injured, defiled, or disfigured, first by the dread disease and then by medical treatment. Like a victim of any kind of overwhelming trauma, we become aware that we have been violated, so that our life, our body, and our soul can never again be the same.

Fear can escalate with dizziness, palpitations, shortness of breath, sweating, and other symptoms of a full panic attack. If we think that these symptoms are caused by the cancer rather than just being our body's way of reacting to fear, that thought alone is terrifying.

"How does one kill fear, I wonder?" one of the characters in Joseph Conrad's novel *Lord Jim* asks. "How do you slash a spectre through the heart, slash off its spectral head, take it by its spectral throat?"

Frustration, Anger, Outrage

No man is angry that feels not himself hurt.

Francis Bacon, "On Anger," *Essays*

We feel tricked and betrayed by our body, by God, or by the universe. We did nothing to deserve this and often feel cheated and bitter at the injustice that so much has been taken from our life. There are things we want to do in our lives and we know we might be deprived of doing them. Our feelings of confidence and security, our hopes, our expectations, and our plans all have been betrayed, so we protest. We rage, as the poet Dylan Thomas put it, "against the dying of the light." Our view of the world has been overturned and the result is at times a loss of faith. The universe, we often believe, is not fair and it is supposed to be. We can't help wondering what kind of universe we live in, and we don't like our conclusions. (As Helene, a woman with Hodgkin's disease, put it, "If we're smart, we don't face the big questions of life because once you pick them up you can't put them down. But cancer forces you to face the big questions.") No one deserves this, and the more we understand the injustice done to us, the more outraged we are.

Our anger is easily displaced, almost at random, in all directions. We might be angry at our doctors, sometimes for not returning our calls promptly, or not taking enough time to talk with us, for giving us information that we cannot understand, for giving us information so brutally that it rips away our hopes, or for their apparent indifference to who we are, to our feelings, and to the urgency of our situation. We are angry at them for ordering all kinds of costly tests and administering all kinds of unpleasant treatments. Sometimes we are angry with them because they are supposed to be our saviors and they aren't saving us from our suffering. At times we resent the people closest to us, and even all the healthy people around us because they don't have to deal with all that we do, and they can enjoy all the things that we can't. Even though we know that our anger and irritability are sometimes irrational, we feel that we have no control when we lash out. Sometimes we are angry at the people we love most because they cannot understand what it is like for us. Sometimes we are angry with them because they are well, or because they are powerless to make us better, or because they nag at us to do things they think are good for us. At times we can't stop ourselves from directing our anger at them simply because they are there.

Sometimes we are angry at ourselves because we feel that somehow we let this happen, or because we are ill and cannot control our body, and because we put the people who love us in a terrible situation.

Grief and Sorrow

The grief that does not speak
Whispers the o'erfraught heart and bids it break.
William Shakespeare, *Macbeth*, IV, iii, 20

Beneath our anger is usually grief so profound that it is beyond the scope of language. It is easier and it hurts less to feel anger, resentment, and bitterness than to face the deep underlying sorrow that tears at our heart. We feel crushing anguish, sometimes despair, for all we have lost. We grieve for our health, our strength, our energy, our independence, the body we knew, the self we knew, and the life we had. We mourn for all that has been taken from us, but perhaps most of all for our dreams of the future that we feel might never be fulfilled.

Guilt

At times we blame ourselves because we feel that somehow we must have caused our cancer, or at least that we could have prevented it. We speculate endlessly about how we did this, perhaps by eating a poor diet, smoking, not exercising, or by staying in a stressful relation-ship or job. Sometimes we think that our illness is a punishment for something we did or didn't do, or that someone else is to blame. Very often we feel guilty for all the pain we are causing the people who love and care for us, and the many burdens we are placing on them.

Our guilt makes our burden heavier. It makes it harder for us to deal with everything and everyone, and leads us to hopelessness.

Hopelessness and Despair

In a real dark night of the soul it is always three o'clock in the morning, day after day.

F. Scott Fitzgerald, *The Crack-Up*

Whether in pain or not, at times we are unable to imagine that any-thing will change, except perhaps for the worse. We feel cheated. We believe that the way things look to us now is the way they will always be, as if we are on a winding road with no exits. Our hopelessness might stem from our feeling of isolation, from pain, or from depres-sion. Perhaps it emerges from our belief that there is no treatment that will help us, or our feeling that neither the people we know nor our physicians really understand or care. Whatever its source, at times each day does indeed feel to us like the darkest night of our soul.

Isolation and Loneliness

In his writings about his experience with cancer during the last months of his life, literary critic Anatole Broyard spoke of "the loneliness of the critically ill, a solitude as haunting as a Chirico painting" (1992, p. 42).

Whatever the severity of our condition, cancer shatters our feeling of connection with others. In our illness we are alone with ourselves.

At times we feel a thick wall separating us from all the people who are healthy, a wall between ourselves and the world of life, movement, and open expectations. Tolstoy, describing a man with cancer in *The Death of Ivan Ilyich*, wrote, "In the bosom of his family, Ivan was so alone he could have been at the bottom of the sea or on the other side of the moon."

Sometimes we deal with all that is happening by withdrawing. We want and need desperately for others to understand what it is like for us. Even so, at times we don't want to talk about how we feel. We realize all too clearly that our illness is not self-contained but extends outward to those closest to us, but this realization can cause us to feel even more isolated. Sometimes we don't talk because we know we will not be understood. At times we just don't want to talk. Language seems insignificant, and besides, our experience cannot be shaped into words. Sometimes we think that our thoughts are too terrible to express. If we are feeling sick, there are times when talking seems to be not worth all the effort and is the last thing we want to do. What we want at those times from those around us is simply respect for our desire to be silent about what is going on with us. Our silence, however, can immobilize us further. We often feel conflicted between wanting to be left alone and yet wanting the comfort of close human contact.

Often there are overtones of devastation and desolation, particularly because the world outside us is unscathed. As if nothing extraordinary has happened, people go about their usual business of living, children play, the sun continues to rise, and the postman delivers mail. Brueghel's plowman, staring intently at the furrows of the earth, takes no notice that Icarus is falling from the sky. Life continues as if we were never a part of it (Ascher, 1993). Our devastation is far more than just a passing emotion. We are strangers in a strange world, the underworld of sickness.

Books about cancer do not usually mention that a cancer diagnosis and the experience of dealing with it is a psychological trauma, nor are many health professionals aware of this. Like a victim of any kind of overwhelming psychic trauma, we feel, at least initially, that our world has split apart abruptly from under us and the sky has tilted. We feel bewildered, vulnerable, and fragile, perhaps as never before. Sometimes we lose our belief that life has any meaning. Whatever else we might feel, we also feel stalked, even haunted—by cancer, death, and dread.

In *Trauma and Recovery*, which deals with reactions to all kinds of atrocities, from war to rape, captivity, and abuse (but not life-threatening illnesses), Judith Lewis Herman writes:

> In situations of terror, people spontaneously seek their first source of comfort and protection. Wounded soldiers cry for their mothers, or for God. When their cry is not answered, their sense of basic trust is shattered. Traumatized people feel utterly abandoned, utterly alone, cast out of the human and divine system of care and protection that sustains life. Therefore, a sense of alienation, of disconnectedness pervades every relationship. . . . When trust is lost, traumatized people feel they belong more to the dead than the living. (1992, p. 52)

Pain

When pain takes hold, our lack of connection is even greater. In the loud loneliness of our pain we are in fact alone, for no one can feel it with us. The 19th-century French novelist Alphonse Daudet described the isolation of a painful illness in his book *Pain* (translated into English as *In the Land of Pain*). He wrote, "There is no general theory of pain. Each person discovers his own. . . . Pain is always new to the sufferer, but loses its originality for those around him. Everyone will get used to it except me" (2002, pp. 15, 19).

Nothing is more real, more certain, more immediate to the sufferer than physical pain, even while it is invisible to others and incommunicable. Physical pain keeps us in the immediate present. If it is agonizing, it portends something worse (Goldie, 2005). Our awareness of our body as the physical basis of our being is blurred when pain obliterates all but the area of the overwhelming sensations. In pain we are reduced to the helplessness and dependency of our childhood.

Pain is alien and incomprehensible. The kind of pain healthy people are familiar with is a signal, a warning, telling us that something is wrong and what to do. The pain of touching a hot stove, for example, warns us to draw back. Chronic or extreme pain, however, has no reference outside of our body and does not tell us how to act. Because it does not appear to follow from who we are, what we have done, it seems to be utterly senseless. We try to make sense of it, so we assign causes, but sometimes when we do our old guilts and anxieties are aroused because we think of it as punishment, retribution for something we have done (LeShan, 1964).

When the pain is overwhelming or apparently without end, when its source is unknown or its meaning is dire, we feel it as a threat to our continued existence—not just to our lives but to our integrity as persons (LeShan, 1964).

Loss of Self

Disease makes men more physical; it leaves them nothing but body.

Thomas Mann, *The Magic Mountain*

With cancer we lose confidence in our bodies and our powers. (Steve, a client of mine, remarked that his body had come to be "a separate thing" from him.) We lose what we now recognize to have been our illusion of safety. We lose the healthy, energetic person we used to be, and feel that we are unable to lose anything more. Suddenly we find ourselves diminished: vulnerable, bewildered, and insecure, helpless in many ways, in a world we do not know. The treatment might have produced physical changes that we feel can devastate our life. Men treated for cancer of the testicle might feel castrated. Women who have had a breast removed or have been made infertile after treatment for cancer of the reproductive organs might feel that they are no longer women. People who have had surgery on their larynx, esophagus, or tongue have lost their main means of communication (Goldie, 2005). People with ostomy surgery feel that their bodies have become deformed.

Our loss of independence and inability to do what we always do can make us feel worthless. If cancer changes the things about ourselves on which we base our feelings of worth, we can easily lose our self-esteem. Because we are weak and dependent, feeling sick, tired, and perhaps in pain, sometimes unable to take care of ourselves in basic ways, incapable of carrying out our normal roles, routines, and responsibilities, we feel inadequate. At times there is no way for us to act; we can only try to bear what is happening. This passivity makes it even harder for us to feel and act like ourselves. Our experience seems impossible to accept, communicate, and integrate. Because our bodies seem out of control, because we can't function normally, and because our entire life has been overturned by our illness and treatments, we often feel that we don't know who we are.

We are accustomed to seeing ourselves as part of a familiar pattern of life. Now the pattern has been ripped apart and our life has become incoherent. We are accustomed to having many roles in our lives: spouse, parent, child, friend, colleague, worker, lover of all the things we choose to do and the people we want to be with. All those roles are diminished, overshadowed by another: We have become a cancer patient. People treat us as if we are cancer with a person attached rather than a person with cancer, and we come to feel this way. We feel ourselves to be nothing but our illness. Cancer and cancer treatment take over our life and our identity.

We lose our goals and purposes, and as we do our inner life decays. The psychiatrist Viktor Frankl wrote, "It is a peculiarity of man that he can only live by looking to the future" (1959, p. 74). But when we are in emotional or physical pain, we are pulled to the immediate present.

If we can see no future, all too often we see ourselves as sick patients in a situation that will never change. Our sense of self, of all that we are, is blurred and sometimes lost to us. We feel a sense of terrible emptiness, as if we have lost our soul. At times in the loud silence and loneliness of our illness, only our existence is real. Without gravity we float alone in space, too often conscious only of our suffering.

If you have never been in this situation, try to imagine it: Your world has capsized, the pattern of your life is fragmented, and there is no rescue. Even if you are not in pain or disfigured from treatment, you feel that you can neither live in the present nor plan for the future. Cancer seems to have permeated everything. Your images of yourself, the life you know, your relationships, and your sense of trust are all diminished, clouded, and confused. You are drained, crushed, with no more energy left. Nothing is the same and you fear that it never will be. You feel you have lost the body and the self you knew, your vitality, and your future, and you will not know for a long time whether you are to return to life. The people around you, no matter how much they love you, don't seem to understand what it's like for you, and you don't know how to put it into words. You can't explain that you're burning out. You feel like you have been in a shipwreck and are lost, trying to stay afloat when neither you nor those around you know how you can keep from drowning. At times you get so tired that you aren't at all sure how long you can continue to try.

These are the dark emotional symptoms of cancer and treatment. They are natural human responses to the traumatic situation that these people are trying to handle—but they are not the only ones. Very often they go hand in hand with strength, integrity, love, courage, and determination to fight for life.

CHAPTER 9

Choosing Practitioners and Treatments, and Communicating With Doctors

The family is only a team when every member joins in the making of decisions. The patient especially needs to feel in control. It is after all, the patient's life that is on the line.

Stephanie Mathews Simonton,
The Healing Family (1989, p. 51)

The most difficult time for someone with cancer and the family is the period between the diagnosis until shortly after treatment begins. The diagnosis usually leaves everyone in the family feeling overwhelmed and confused, unable to comprehend fully what is happening and what it means. Once decisions have been made and treatment has begun, the initial emotional tempest usually lessens. Instead of catastrophic fantasies about what the treatment is like, the patient experiences the reality, finds he can live with it, and thus regains some sense of control. However, to get from the storm to relative calm, a number of critical decisions must be made. The patient and family are usually faced with more medical alternatives than they usually expect, and are ill equipped to make good choices about doctors and treatments.

Perhaps their psychological situation can best be conveyed metaphorically. Imagine that you are standing on soft ground that is sinking. In front of you are two or more doors, and you have to go through one of them. One might kill you and one might save your life, but you don't know which. Your most trusted advisors don't agree—and you have to make a decision because the ground is giving way beneath your feet. Imagine how you would feel.

Such decisions are stressful and frightening, for they will have a profound effect on the lives of everyone involved. To add to their stress, many people fear conventional cancer treatments. They think of them only as drastic solutions with harmful effects. For that reason, numerous patients turn to unproven cancer therapies, often with tragic consequences. It is important for patients and family members to understand that conventional medicine for cancer facilitates the body's own self-healing ability. That is, in one way or another, conventional treatments aim at destroying or weakening malignant cells. In so doing, they increase the body's own ability to heal from an illness that could otherwise be fatal. In the process of saving the patient's life, to be sure, some treatments might cause side effects or aftereffects. Normal cells might be damaged, but when this happens they are then replaced by new cells. Some normal cells damaged by treatment might not be replaced, but usually in that case remaining cells take over their function. When the body is injured or damaged in any way by treatment, the body's self-healing abilities begin the process of repair.

Gathering medical information in order to choose treatments and doctors is among the most important things patients and families can do. Unlike many other illnesses, for many forms of cancer there is no one best treatment. Combinations of treatments are usually recommended, and the precise mix often varies from one physician to another. Different treatments have different results and different side effects. For that reason, physicians usually suggest several treatment options and explain their expected outcomes and effects.

The way to begin is with information. It is important that the patient and family be encouraged to learn at least basic facts and concepts about the disease and available treatment options. By so doing, they can communicate better with their physicians, participate in making medical decisions, make more informed choices, and better handle medical care. Further, from a number of studies it has become very clear that patients who take charge from the outset get the best results and have the best quality of life. Being in charge, however, does not mean doing everything. This chapter provides some guidelines for taking charge.

Gathering Information About the Diagnosis

Whether cancer is discovered during a routine physical examination or when the patient has consulted the primary physician or an internist after experiencing symptoms, it is this doctor who takes responsibility for the diagnosis. The physician might refer the patient to an oncologist, a physician specializing in cancer treatment, or a surgeon. Different oncologists specialize in treating different kinds of cancer. Surgical oncologists specialize in surgery, medical oncologists in chemotherapy treatments, and radiation oncologists in radiation treatments.

More than one test procedure might be necessary, so it might take days or even weeks to get the final diagnosis. During that time, the patient and family often go back and forth between the anxiety of waiting to learn the test results and the feeling that they don't want to know. This is the beginning of their experience of living with not knowing what is going to happen, perhaps one of the most difficult places for anyone to be.

News of the diagnosis usually comes from the primary physician who receives the test results. It is difficult to imagine anyone who does not react with shock and fear, along with other typical reactions (described in chapters 1 and 8). However, despite these responses, it is essential that the patient seek medical information and help. People diagnosed with cancer who reject the diagnosis—for example, by refusing to believe it, by not talking about it, by not seeking medical help, by refusing medical treatment, or by seeking out questionable practitioners or treatments—are needlessly putting their lives in great danger.

At this time, or during another appointment soon afterward, the patient and family members need to obtain basic information. Clearly, the more information the family has about the patient's specific kind of cancer, the more control they can take. (General information about cancer and diagnoses can be found in Appendix 1.)

Family members can be of enormous help by gathering information about the patient's condition from the doctor, from books and articles, and from the Internet. Many Internet sites provide cancer information, but not all the information on the Web is safe and trustworthy. The most credible are those sponsored by health organizations such as the American Cancer Society, by the government, and by major medical institutions such as Harvard, Stanford, the Mayo Clinic, and Johns Hopkins University.

From the physician, patients and family members need the following information about test results and diagnoses:

- What is the diagnosis—the type and stage of the tumor?
- Where is the tumor located—in which area or organ?
- What is the size of the tumor?
- Has it spread? If so, to where?
- How fast does it appear to be growing?
- What kind of tests led to the diagnosis? (Fiore, 1990)

At this point, the physician might refer the family to an oncologist or surgeon to discuss treatment options.

Gathering Information About Treatment Options

The patient and family would do well to try to learn as much as possible about the various treatment options suggested, beginning with their expected beneficial effects. Any cancer treatment is expected to serve one of three purposes: to cure the cancer, to slow or arrest it to extend the patient's life, or to improve the quality of life so that the patient is fairly pain-free and symptom-free for as long as possible.

Acquiring information about treatment options is important. However, for many forms of cancer, there is not always just one clear-cut best treatment. Specialists consulted are likely to offer more than one alternative for the kind of cancer the patient has. Different physicians might disagree, and some might be indecisive or offer more than option. Because there is no one best treatment for cancer, no physician can advise about a definitive treatment, so that these decisions are difficult and frightening. One of the many things patients and families have to deal with is the unsettling lack of certainty they encounter.

There are three primary conventional treatments, used singly or in combination: surgery to remove all or part of the tumor, radiation to disable cancer cells, and chemotherapy to shrink or destroy the tumor with certain kinds of drugs. It can be of great help to the patient if family members handle much or all of the research about treatment options. (Basic information about these and other treatments can be found in Appendix 2.)

From the specialist, patients and family members need the following information:

- What are the treatment options?
- What are the goals of each?
- What treatment plan does this physician recommend, and why?
- If the proposed treatment has several components, what is the rationale for their sequence?
- What are the expected outcomes or benefits of the treatment (or each treatment component)?
- What are the chances of improvement?
- What are the risks?
- What are the likely short- and long-term side effects? Are there ways to decrease side effects?
- What quality of life can be expected after treatment?

- How is the treatment administered?
- What are the risks of doing nothing?
- What recommendations can this doctor make for a second opinion?
- What can the patient do to improve her health? (Anderson, 1999; Fiore, 1990; LeVert, 1995; Simonton, 1984)

Getting a Second Opinion

Second opinions have saved many lives. Unless the patient's condition requires treatment urgently, anyone with a life-threatening illness should get another opinion, whatever the prognosis.

Many people are inclined not to question their doctors and to accept their recommendations implicitly. However, doctors and pathologists can make mistakes. Each physician is likely to have had more experience with some kinds of cancer and some treatments than others, and accuracy differs from one facility or practitioner to another. What is at least as important is that different doctors have different attitudes about treatment. Some are most interested in eradicating the cancer and so might recommend aggressive treatment, regardless of many side effects. Others are most interested in the quality of the patient's life and so might take a more cautious approach by recommending treatments that are less harsh. Before agreeing to treatment, every cancer patient deserves to have the first opinion confirmed and other options explored. Without a qualified second opinion, treatment possibilities are limited from the start (Anderson, 1999; Fiore, 1990).

The purpose of another opinion is not to learn whether cancer is in fact present or the diagnosis incorrect. It is to get an independent confirmation of the first physician's account of it, and other treatment recommendations. Different doctors have different ideas and attitudes about what constitutes the best treatment, and it is important to get more than one viewpoint (Fiore, 2000).

The second opinion needs to come from a well-qualified, board-certified specialist, usually an oncologist, experienced in the precise kind of cancer and problems the patient has. The specialist consulted should be in a different practice from the first physician, trained separately, and working in a different treatment center or hospital, or even in a different city or state.

Physicians often advise patients that cancer treatment should begin as soon as possible. The time the cancer is discovered is the time when a number of options may be viable, so it is the time for decision making. However, few kinds of cancer constitute an emergency. No one should be rushed into neglecting to take the time to get another opinion. After all, the effects of some treatments, particularly some kinds of surgery, cannot be reversed. If the first doctor consulted discourages another opinion, that is reason enough to seek one.

Family members and patients should not be concerned with offending their doctor by saying they want another opinion. Even if the patient and family members like and trust the first doctor, talking to another specialist in the patient's kind of cancer is never a waste of time. There are constantly new developments in cancer treatments, and it is difficult for every doctor to keep abreast of all of them. Getting a second opinion is not a luxury but standard procedure. Some insurers will not reimburse for treatment without one. Other insurers might not provide reimbursement for another opinion, but with the patient's life at stake it is well worth the cost.

The patient and family should not hesitate to tell the first physician that they intend to get another opinion, not simply as a matter of courtesy, but also so that the doctor can send copies of necessary records (including slides, scans, X-rays, case write-ups) to the doctor they plan to see. Good doctors will not be threatened by a patient asking to see another specialist. Years ago doctors did not typically advise their patients to seek a second opinion, but today most good physicians encourage it.

An appropriate practitioner for a consultation can be found in university medical centers, large teaching hospitals, comprehensive cancer treatment canters, or in a private practice. Information about qualified physicians can be had from national cancer societies, medical associations, local hospitals, or from the primary physician.

Treatment for most kinds of cancer is based on what has been shown to be most effective. Each physician will probably consider the statistically preferred treatment and also offer alternatives. The second opinion might agree with the first and validate it. In this case, it will bring the patient and family peace of mind to learn that both doctors concur. If the two recommendations are not consistent, there are two options. Assuming that both specialists are highly qualified, the family might decide that either physician's approach might constitute excellent care. Alternately, they might decide to seek a third opinion.

Seeking a third opinion is a perfectly reasonable course to take if they are not sure that the opinions they have do not constitute the best or only treatment choices. It is surely the best course to take if the recommendations they already have are not consistent. Seeking a third or a fourth opinion is not a reasonable course to take if the purpose is to shop for doctors with the hope of finding one who says what the family wants to hear. Rather, the purpose of another opinion is to arrive at what the patient is confident is the best possible treatment plan. However, to travel all over the country to seek out many different opinions is not only financially wasteful but wasteful of time that can better be spent beginning a treatment. Two opinions that agree are usually adequate.

The family, including the patient to the greatest extent possible, should be encouraged to continue to gather information, consult experts, and reflect on their own attitude about treatment until they can arrive at clarity and conviction about a doctor and a treatment plan. If they understand the treatment, the need for it, and its possible side effects, it is not something mysterious that is forced on the patient.

When treatment decisions have been made, there is other information that the patient and family need in order to make plans:

• When can the patient expect to be able to resume work and family responsibilities?
• During the treatment period, what activities and responsibilities can the patient be expected to handle?

- What kind of help is likely to be needed—for example, with household chores, child care, and travel to and from the treatment center?

Cancer treatment is physically and psychologically difficult for anyone. The going is likely to get rough, and when it does and patients feel sick or in pain, even though they know the purpose of their treatment, they might become resistant to continuing with it. ("I know I have to and I should, but I don't want any more.") Because of this predictable ambivalence, it is important that patients be given time to make treatment decisions. Patients are under far less strain when they understand the treatment, the need for it, its possible side effects, and its benefits. What is wanted is that they commit to the treatment, not just submit to it. This can happen only if they fully understand their options, discuss them with their physicians and families, make their choices, and then feel confident that their decision is the best one for them. If this does not happen, the experience they will have, as well as their adjustment and recovery, will be far more difficult (American Cancer Society and CURE, 2008; Anderson, 1999; Balch, 2008; Fiore, 1990).

Integrative Medicine

Based on the findings of years of mind-body research, an increasing number of physicians offer or recommend an integrative ("holistic") treatment approach involving the use of complementary (adjunctive") therapies in addition to conventional medical treatments. More and more cancer patients are seeking out such therapies, whether their physicians recommend them or not. (These therapies are *not* alternatives to standard medical treatments, but used in conjunction with them.) While medical treatments target the cancer, complementary therapies treat the whole person by strengthening the full range of the patient's self-healing resources and improving physical and mental health.

They include individualized nutritional programs, psychotherapy, yoga, massage, visualization, and meditation, and spiritual modalities.

(Appendix 2 includes a description of these and other adjunctive modalities.)

No one therapy or any combination of conventional and complementary treatments can guarantee a cure. However, patients and family members would be well advised to learn about available complementary options, particularly an individualized nutritional program, for patients to consider and explore. There is good reason to believe that these therapies not only improve patients' quality of life, but, because of their improved physical and mental strength, help them to become more resilient to medical treatments—and perhaps even to the illness itself. (Lerner, 1998)

Choosing Doctors

Conventional cancer treatment is provided by a group of physicians that includes an oncologist and often also a surgeon or radiation oncologist. The patient will also be treated by other practitioners they do not select who will be involved in different aspects of care, such as other surgeons, radiology technicians, or oncology nurses. One of the physicians, usually the oncologist, will be the one heading the team. Specialists can be found at large community hospitals, cancer treatment centers, university medical complexes, or in private practice.

The specialist consulted for a second or third opinion might not be the one to treat the patient. For example, many patients seek expert opinions in major cancer centers or in hospitals known for treating their kind of cancer in another city, and then select physicians locally to administer treatment. The choice of a medical team is as important as the choice of treatment, so families should be encouraged to choose their physicians very carefully.

Every patient has the right to be treated by practitioners who are knowledgeable, skilled, and experienced. The first consideration needs to be the doctor's credentials and expertise in the field of specialization. Treating physicians should be board-certified specialists in the type of cancer the patient has, and should have worked for at least a few years in the field. The patient and family will want to inquire about the doctor's training, experience, philosophy, and fee structure.

Another consideration is simply convenience. If the patient is to have radiation, which is administered daily, or frequent chemotherapy, a physician working in a facility located nearby is desirable.

Every patient also has the right to be treated by practitioners who are compassionate, caring, and encouraging. Once it is established that the physician is qualified and experienced, families need to encourage patients to trust their responses to the practitioner as a human being. While competence is the first consideration, the physician's attitude about the patient and the patient's future is the second. The patient needs to feel that the doctor genuinely cares and is someone the patient likes and feels she can trust. Hope influences the patient's quality of life and even recovery. It is unlikely that anyone can sustain hope if the treating physician conveys hopelessness.

Traditionally physicians have been viewed as the ultimate authorities on patients' illness and healing, while patients are passive recipients. In recent years this view has changed: The physician-patient relationship is seen more and more as a partnership. The physician's job is to bring to the patient the best that medical science has to offer and to engage the emotional resources of the patient to the fullest. The patient brings self-healing abilities that can be activated by a strong will to live and powerful expectations of recovery (Cousins, 1986).

For this reason, doctors' personalities, attitudes, and relationships with their patients are as important as their expertise. This is particularly important when it comes to oncologists and any others whom the patient will be seeing most often. It is far less important when it comes to surgeons, who see their patients for a relatively short time, and whose skill and experience are more vital to the patient than bedside manner.

Here are some guidelines to consider:

- Is the physician someone in whom the patient feels trust?
- Does the physician seem interested in the patient as an individual, not just as a case?
- Does the physician treat the patient with respect and understanding?
- Does the physician sccm caring, warm, and sensitive (rather than authoritarian and remote)?
- Does the doctor relate to the patient as a competent adult?
- Does the doctor try to consider the patient's psychological and emotional as well as physical needs?
- Is the patient comfortable being and talking with the physician?
- Does the doctor encourage the patient to ask questions?
- Does the physician listen?
- Is the physician open to input from the patient about symptoms, treatment, and options?
- Does the physician take the time to answer questions in a way that is easy to understand?
- Does the physician appear to appreciate that cancer is confusing and frightening, and respond with patience and kindness to the patient's concerns?
- Does the physician leave the patient reassured and hopeful about the outcome?
- Does the doctor instill a feeling of confidence and security?
- Is the doctor accepting of family members' involvement?
- Does the doctor give the patient undivided attention during each visit and spend adequate time?
- Is the physician available on the telephone and, in case of emergencies, on weekends?
- Does the physician return phone calls?
- Can appointments be made fairly soon after they are requested or needed?
- Is the physician on time for appointments?

Apart from their medical competence, doctors relate to their patients in different ways. Some create a personal connection with their patients and are warm and gentle; others are direct, impersonal, distant, and unemotional. Some physicians are sensitive to their patients' emotional needs, while others brutally rip away their hopes. When it comes to medical decisions, some physicians encourage a partnership with patients, while others relate to patients as authoritarian parents. If the patient is not confident or comfortable with the doctor, the question should be considered as to whether it might be in the patient's best interests to look elsewhere until he finds a physician he feels is the right one.

It needs to be stressed that while it is enormously important that family members be involved, it is the patient who is in charge of medical treatment and care and who needs to make treatment decisions. Families sometimes believe that they will be helping by making treatment decisions without the patient's involvement, but this belief is completely misguided. The patient's way of handing difficult decisions may be different from that of the family, and the patient's decisions might be different from what family members want. However, the patient's style and choices must be respected. In any case, few physicians will proceed without the full understanding and consent of the patient. Again, studies have shown that when patients participate in their care and are committed to their treatment, they fare better medically and also recover more quickly. This is far more likely to happen when they understand the long-term benefits of a treatment that might well have undesirable side effects in the short term.

Patients' beliefs and attitudes make a difference to their survival, so the family needs to continue keeping their options open. There is no reason to stay with a doctor with whom the patient is uncomfortable, or whom the patient does not trust. Nor is there any reason to stay with a physician whose attitude works against the patient's hope. People who have recovered from cancer have expressed their conviction that there is a direct correlation between their confidence in their doctors and their recovery. What is wanted is a group of physicians and a treatment plan the patient believes in. It is a mistake to settle for less (Alpha Institute, 1998).

Communicating With Doctors

The medical situation has changed in recent years. Most people can no longer consult one doctor for all their needs. Most doctors, even those specializing in internal medicine, refer patients to specialists for diagnoses and follow-up care. They no longer have the training and expertise to perform the kinds of test needed, many of which have been developed in recent years. They also have less time than to spend with each patient than in the past. Patients are different, too. They tend to be more knowledgeable about their illnesses.

Oncologists, surgeons, and radiation oncologists are experts in cancer treatment, trained to think in terms of human bodies. However, there is far more to any patient than her cancer and her body. As individuals, patients are the only world experts on themselves. Doctors are not mind readers. When it comes to any patient, they cannot know everything or always know best. Open communication between patients and their physicians is a vital aspect of cancer treatment. It is the responsibility of patients to play an active role in their treatment. One way is to communicate their needs and concerns so as to get what they need from each medical visit.

Receiving Information

Patients need as much or as little information as they want. It is important that they tell their physician how much they want to know. (For example, do they want to know the statistical odds of survival or what to expect if the cancer progresses?) Physicians can be expected to provide basic information about test results and about the illness and treatment. Beyond this, however, they have to be told what information is wanted. Otherwise they cannot know what is going on with their patients, what their patients are afraid of, and what they want to know. Most patients do not want to hear bad news, and physicians may be unlikely to volunteer it.

People vary as to the amount of information about the illness and treatment they want. Some want all the information they can get. For them, not knowing is frightening. Others do not want to know all the details. For them, knowing is more frightening. Doctors have no way of knowing what or how much information patients want about their illness, and so may not provide certain kinds of information unless they are asked.

However much or little information the patient wants, it is helpful for family members to learn all they can about the illness and treatment, so they can better help the patient during treatment. Family members might want information that the patient does not want to know, such as the likely ramifications of treatment. For these reasons, it is extremely helpful if the patient and family members clarify to themselves early on what information they want from doctors, and then discuss how they want this information handled.

Any questions family members have for the doctors should be asked in the presence of the patient. (In other words, it is not a good idea for a relative to follow the doctor down the hall to ask questions that the patient cannot hear.) In any case, the physician's primary responsibility is to the patient, not the family. Physicians will provide information to them only if the patient authorizes them to do so.

It is helpful for the family to assign one person to talk with the doctor when the patient is unable to do so. It should be someone the patient trusts and who communicates clearly. This person will be the one to ask the physician questions when necessary and disseminate information to the patient and others in the family, and whom the doctor can call in case of emergency (Babcock, 1997).

Even before treatment starts, the patient's and family's relationship with the doctor begins. Family members can help the patient with medical appointments by facilitating communication. Patients are understandably anxious during their doctor appointments and might not be able to listen well or retain information. It is advisable that someone always accompany the patient to see the doctor, to listen, and to take notes or tape record what the doctor says. The patient can plan to make the most of the appointment time by preparing a list of written questions.

Providing Information, Asking Questions, Airing Concerns

Some patients believe that once they have agreed to a treatment, they must simply bear any unpleasant side effects. It is helpful to remember that the physician is there not only to deal with the illness, but to help with patients' problems and concerns. To receive the best possible care, it is vital that patients ask for what they want: more information, a test, an examination, or different medications.

To this end, it is advisable that patients prepare a list of information and questions. This list should include anything causing the patient anxiety, pain, or discomfort: symptoms, their frequency, their severity, when they began, and how they are inferring with the patient's life. It is wise to list these in order of priority so that at least the most pressing ones will be dealt with, and to make sure that each item on the list is stated clearly. Such a list can also help to ensure that appointment times are not wasted with off-track questions. To best help the doctor help them, patients should make an effort to communicate their problems, wishes, and concerns as clearly and factually as possible, without either minimizing or exaggerating.

The physician's viewpoint about treatment may not include complementary approaches. Besides providing information about symptoms and reactions, patients need to inform their physician about any forms of complementary treatment they are using, particularly diet and supplements. They should prepare a list of any nonprescription herbs and vitamins they are taking, along with other medications, dosages, and frequency of use.

If the doctor says or recommends anything that the patient or family member does not understand, it is important to speak up and ask for clarification. ("Would you please explain this in plain language?")

If the doctor provides any written material that the patient or family member is unsure about, it is important to get help in understanding it. ("This looks like it might be hard to understand." "Do you have anything that is easier to read?" "Whom can we call if there is something we don't understand?")

Otherwise, the patient might not follow recommendations because information was misunderstood. In particular, it is vital that the patient understand what medications are being prescribed and what they are for.

If the doctor suggests or recommends anything without explaining the reason for it, it is also important for the patient speak up about this, to ask and, if necessary, continue to ask until the information is understood. If the doctor does anything or communicates in a way that the patient has a problem with, it is important to ask about this, too. Even if the patient and family members believe they understand what they have told, they can make sure that they do. ("I think I understand, but let me make sure by telling you what I heard.")

Besides physical problems, the patient should understand that it is appropriate to bring up any emotional, physical, and sexual concerns and fears. Patients who are open with their doctors about their fears and feelings are likely to get the same level of openness in return (Simonton, 1984).

Common Complaints

Patients have some common complaints:

- The physician does not spend enough time with them.
- They are treated inconsiderately or impersonally.
- The physician discourages a complementary treatment that the patient believes is helpful.
- The physician makes recommendations without explaining them.
- The physician does not inform them of all their medical options.
- The physician does not provide information they can understand.
- The physician does not take the time to answer questions.
- The physician does not involve them in decisions about their care.

If patients find that their physician does not spend enough time with them, the next time they schedule an appointment they can ask for some extra time for questions. ("Doctor, I have more questions.") Some patients mail, fax, or e-mail a brief note to their physicians prior to their appointment to state concerns they would like to discuss.

If patients feel that the physician is treating them impersonally or inconsiderately, they can say so. ("Doctor, it's very difficult for me to sit and wait for you for 2 or 3 hours, and I'm not willing to do that again. What can we do about this?") If they feel the doctor is treating them only as a case and ignoring them as whole individuals, they can make it clear that their emotional well-being is as vital to them as their medical treatment. They can also explain that they will take responsibility for helping to make this happen.

If they feel that the physician is not providing adequate information, it is up to patients to assert that they want to participate in treatment decisions and that they need information to do so.

Another common complaint is that physicians take away their hope. In this case, patients can express this. As one of my clients put it to her oncologist, "I need you to be positive." Her physician heard her and responded immediately. If he hadn't, she would have sought another doctor.

When physicians do not respond to complaints, concerns, questions, and requests, their patients' confidence in them erodes. For example, when patients feel that their doctor is not informing them of all their medical options, not providing adequate information, or not treating them as partners in their own care, this engenders mistrust. Confidence in the physician affects patients' attitudes and their responses to treatment. Without it, there is no reason to stay with that physician. A lack of trust in their source of care only causes more suffering. When a physician does not make a patient feel comfortable or refuses to give the patient any hope, this, too, can strongly affect the patient's state of mind and response to treatment. If patients do not trust or have faith in their doctor, they would do well to request and seek a different doctor.

The Relationship

The quality of a patient's relationship with physicians is extremely important. A good relationship enhances any patient's quality of life and increases chances of recovery. A bad relationship can impede recovery and also makes life more difficult for everyone involved. Herbert Benson, MD, author of *The Relaxation Response*, wrote that the body's ability to heal itself works best when three elements are present: "One, the belief and expectation of the patient; two, the belief and expectation of the physician; and three, *the interaction of the patient and physician*" (quoted in Benjamin, 1987, p. 173).

Most physicians are caring people, but there are some who are remote, who unknowingly take away the patient's hopes, who don't answer questions, or who treat the patient like a not-very-bright child. Fortunately such doctors are the exception. A doctor who acts and talks in an uncaring or insensitive way, depriving the patient of all hope, is not aware of the critical importance of the relationship with the patient.

It is the responsibility of physicians to instill confidence and a sense of security in their patients, while not being distant or authoritarian. This is not always easy. Many cancer patients and their families are angry at the cancer, and their anger can easily land on the physician. Hopefully an experienced practitioner has learned to expect this kind of reaction and has learned how to give information to patients and families who are frightened and confused in an accurate way that is also supportive and positive.

If the relationship becomes unsatisfactory to the patient, it can be extremely helpful to initiate a discussion with the physician about the expectations of each of them. The discussion can range from how treatment decisions will be made to whether or not to be on a first-name basis. Since every patient is different, the doctor might also welcome such a talk to clarify the relationship.

Responsibilities

As partners in their care, patients also have responsibilities. Meeting those responsibilities greatly helps their relationships with their physicians. These responsibilities naturally include adhering to the agreed treatment plan, as well as keeping appointments on time, being considerate of the doctor's need to spend time with other patients, and being courteous and appreciative to the physician and the staff. Beyond this, however, patients have other responsibilities:

1. To ask for information they want, but without knowingly taking the doctor's time with questions an associate can answer
2. To make sure that they understand all medical information and instructions
3. To be sure they are informed about their medical procedures and treatments
4. To communicate to the physician clearly and directly their wishes, thoughts, and needs, as well as any relevant information such as nutritional programs they are following

Once a physician is selected, the patient and family need to respect that practitioner's view. Healing, however, involves a person's total being: physical, mental, emotional, creative, relational, and whatever that means to the patient, spiritual. It is the doctor's responsibility to take care of the patient's physical body. The rest is up to patients and those close to them.

CHAPTER 10

How Family Caregivers Can Best Help the Cancer Patient

There's no vocabulary
For love within a family, love that's lived in
But not looked at, love within the light of which
All other love finds speech.
This love is silent.

T. S. Eliot, *The Elder Statesman* (1964)

When the initial crisis of a cancer diagnosis becomes an ongoing illness, no one in the family is prepared. Most family members have not been taught how to be caregivers any more than the person who is ill knows how to be a cancer patient. At the same time that family members are dealing with their own fear and confusion about their new situation, they must learn to manage practical and logistical matters involving medical care and everyday living. Whether out of love, devotion, loyalty, obligation, or a combination of these, they want to help.

Family members can contribute to the patient's emotional health and physical recovery in many ways. The patient might accept some and reject others, but love, support, and empathy are almost always welcome.

One family member wrote, "Being the primary caregiver for my brother, I consciously and unconsciously assumed many roles. At various points I felt like a nurse and doctor, counselor and friend, care team manager, and insurance specialist and banker. I was the executor of his estate and had medical and financial powers of attorney. In the end, I found out that the most important thing I could be was just his brother" (Sweeney, 2000, p. 44).

This chapter is about the most important things family members can be for the person who is ill.

Being Present

From the first medical appointment through the last treatment, family members can be there with the patient. To anyone with cancer, knowing that they are not alone and that others want to be there with them through their entire frightening journey is vitally important.

During medical appointments family members can act as extra listeners and, if necessary, provide information if the patient is unable to do so. While they should be with the patient primarily to listen and not to intrude with their own concerns and opinions, their presence can be extremely helpful. After the appointment, they can discuss their understanding of what the doctor said.

Another important consideration is that family members who accompany the patient to treatments are helpful only if they offer more than just their physical presence. Cancer treatments are stressful for patients and caring emotional support is needed.

Tina's husband, Frank, drove her to her chemotherapy treatments every 3 weeks, waited for her, and drove her home. She said, "He acts as if he is just doing his duty. He's sullen. He doesn't talk much to me during the drive or while we're waiting in the office and doesn't seem interested in anything the doctor says. He actually seems resentful, but insists that he wants to take me to my appointments." After her third treatment, Tina asked a close friend of hers to accompany her instead. Frank seemed relieved when she told him.

There are many ways for family members to be present with the patient. While their physical presence is usually enormously helpful, their emotional presence is at least as important. People who are ill need to know that those closest to them love them, want to understand them, and are with them in every possible way. With their words, actions, and attitudes, family members would do well to express and demonstrate how much the patient means to them.

Being an Advocate for Autonomy

One of the most distressing effects of cancer on patients can be their feeling of the loss of control. They often feel they have lost control of their bodies, their functioning, and their lives, and are helpless to direct the course of their illness. Besides being weakened physically by medical treatment, cancer weakens feelings of worth, competence, and self-esteem.

For this reason, one of the most meaningful ways for family members to help is by encouraging patients to exercise control in every possible way. The more control, independence, and autonomy a patient can maintain or regain, the more hope and confidence she is likely to have about her ability to deal with the illness and to recover.

Debby described to me an experience she had after her cancer diagnosis that she believed marked the turning point in her healing. A close friend of hers led her to the large pond in Central Park and arranged for her to direct a miniature sailboat with a remote con-

trol. She spent hours there and during that time, she said, she re-
gained her sense of control over her life.

That was one effective way for one individual. Encouraging patients to
become informed and involved in medical decisions is another. Family
members can discuss treatment options and their opinions about them
with the patient. Then they can encourage the patient to take the time
to make a considered, informed choice, without feeling pressured by
the family or medical practitioners to make one choice rather than another.

> When Mary was diagnosed with breast cancer, she felt that her
> worst nightmare had come true. For many years, she had been
> afraid of getting breast cancer because her aunt, to whom she had
> been very close, had died years earlier of metastatic cancer origi-
> nating in her breast. Because Mary's tumor was small and the can-
> cer had not spread, her physician advised a lumpectomy (surgical
> removal of the tumor), followed by radiation and chemotherapy.
> Mary, however, believed that her fears could not put to rest unless
> she had her breasts removed. Her husband Brad had been with her
> when the doctor had discussed his recommendations. When they
> left the doctor's office, Brad argued with her, saying that the dou-
> ble mastectomy was a drastic and unnecessary option. The next
> morning, while he still felt strongly that the doctor's proposal was
> the best option, he realized how much he hated the idea of his
> wife losing her breasts. He also realized that no matter what he
> wanted, the decision had to be hers. He told Mary that he loved
> and respected her, and that he would support whatever decision
> she made—and he did.

Some patients are too ill or too frightened to be involved with medical
decisions. They might not be able to handle too much information or
spend time doing research. Feeling like they are under emotional siege,
many people wish that someone else could make medical decisions for

them, and some patients and families just want the comfort of relying on the authority of health care professionals by turning all decisions over to their doctors. Traditionally, patients have been passive, deferring to their doctors and consenting to whatever they advise. Passivity in this situation, however, often does not help. People diagnosed with a life-threatening illness feel that their bodies, as well as their lives, have gone out of control and that they are helpless and might die. Passive compliance with doctors, and even with their family, only heightens that feeling. To lessen these feelings and the resulting despair and depression, patients should be included in deliberation about treatment decisions to whatever extent possible. By acquiring information and becoming actively involved in decision making, they can begin to regain confidence in themselves, and a sense of control as well.

While decisions are best made by patients with the family, it is the patients who need to have the final word. If the family disagrees, the patient's decisions need to be honored. Although the entire family is affected by treatment choices, the patient's life is the one most directly involved. Besides, patients are the only ones who truly know what is going on with them. They know best what they want and how they will adapt to the necessary changes in their lives. When the basic decisions are theirs, they feel more empowered and more confident about the outcome, and they cope better with the treatment. Thus, decision making gives them an essential role to play, as well as an essential responsibility to themselves to maintain their authority with their family and their practitioners.

When a patient is very ill and frail, family members' help is vital to ensure that medical care is adequate. However, patients who are alert and able to be assertive can be expected to advocate for themselves, with little help from family members. Maintaining autonomy is particularly important if patients are in a hospital, where they are expected to comply passively with hospital rules. In that setting, where people are often depersonalized and given little choice even about when to sleep and eat, it is very easy for anyone to feel like a child, a victim, or an anonymous object. In that situation, family members can help by encouraging patients to speak out with any questions or requests about what they want or need.

Family members typically feel the need to do something to help in any way they can. They feel frightened, anxious, and powerless over the illness and seek some kind of control. From their desire to help and to overcome their own feeling of helplessness, a major danger is that they will treat the patient as a child or an invalid. Depriving the patient of independence and authority, however, does psychological harm to the patient and to the family structure as well.

For the sake of patients' emotional and physical well-being, families can be of most help by respecting patients' authority and autonomy, and encouraging their independence. To whatever extent possible, patients need to be in charge not only of health care options but also of everything affecting their life. (After all, people with cancer are ill, not feebleminded.) They should be encouraged to participate as fully as possible in family plans and activities, household tasks, discussions and decisions. Their decisions about themselves should include when to eat and sleep, how to exercise, and what activities to undertake. Even if they are very ill, they should be consulted before the family acts on their behalf. They should have the opportunity to decide about such matters as whether they want to talk with someone who called, whether they want to see someone who wants to visit, and when they want to be alone. They should be asked whether they are up for discussing something that a family member wants to talk about. Decisions about whom to tell about the illness should also be made by the patient in consultation with the family.

Ed, who was on strong chemotherapy, complained that his wife, Fran, nagged him constantly by pushing food on him. Fran complained that Ed wasn't eating enough, that he had to eat more to get well, and that he refused food that she offered. Ed said that he was unable to eat the same foods and amounts that he used to, and that there were some foods he couldn't eat at all. They negotiated, and agreed that Fran would offer food only during regular mealtime and would accept whatever he said. Ed agreed to ask Fran for foods that he felt like eating when he felt like it and to try to keep his nutritional requirements in mind. At the end of the session Fran began to understand that it was Ed, not she, who would be in charge of what he ate or didn't eat.

A different situation might occur. Patients might become dependent in ways that are not necessary. In this case, family members can help most by resisting their temptation to take over tasks that the patient is perfectly capable of handling.

For many years, Mel ran his own business. He worked long hours for his many satisfied clients and as a result was extremely successful. His wife, Anne, worked with him as his secretary. Shortly before his 60th birthday Mel was diagnosed with cancer. He closed his office, had surgery, and began chemotherapy. A few days after each treatment, when he felt well enough for light exercise, he and Anne took a walk after breakfast every morning. Besides taking care of their home, preparing meals, and seeing to his medications, she scheduled all their activities. Whenever it was time to make plans with friends or to set up any kind of appointment, Mel would smile and say, "Talk to my social secretary." Anne arranged everything they did: medical appointments, social visits, evenings out to see films or concerts, and any other activities she could think of that Mel might enjoy. She complained that Mel would make no decisions and took no initiative about anything. When she asked what movie he would like to see, whether he would like to go out for dinner, or what he might like to do, he told her to decide. It was as if after years of shouldering heavy responsibilities in his work, he retired from all further decision making. Mel seemed just to assume that his "social secretary" would take charge of everything, even things he was capable of doing himself. As a result, Anne had little or no time to do things she enjoyed.

She admitted that she was becoming increasingly resentful. After clarifying her feelings, she announced to Mel that she needed time away for herself and that she would like to go out several afternoons each week. She said she would make sure that there was plenty of food in the refrigerator and would put out his medications before she left. She asked him to prepare his own lunches and to take his medications at the right times. Mel seemed surprised that she felt the need to have time by herself, but agreed cheerfully to do what she asked.

Anne's request was reasonable. She was not asking Mel to do more than he could, nor was she expecting too much from him. (If he could take walks, he could make a sandwich, wash his dishes, and take his pills, she figured.) She knew that he was not yet capable of carrying out many more strenuous activities, and did not push him to try to do so.

Besides encouraging the patient to take responsibilities, if family members need something from the person who is ill, they should not hesitate to say so. If something is bothering them, they should not hesitate to speak up. To do otherwise is to regard the patient as an invalid or a helpless child.

Again, the more control and independence patients can exert, the more confident and hopeful they are likely to be. To infantilize them deprives them of feeling responsible and needed, and reinforces their feelings of being victims of their illness.

Joe, who had been diagnosed with gastrointestinal cancer, complained that since his surgery, his wife and his parents had been making personal and business decisions for him without consulting him. He was receiving chemotherapy, and within a week after each treatment, he felt well enough to be able to take care of many of his personal needs. His therapist suggested that he bring his family to his next session. At the scheduled time when everyone was seated, he announced solemnly to the family, "I have some news for all of you. Joe is not dead."

Family caregivers are well advised not to make assumptions about what the patient needs, but rather to ask. Let the patient decide how the family can be supportive of his efforts to function and to get well. The patient might well feel worthless and guilty at being a burden on the family. What can help is to encourage him to be involved in all decisions and allow him to be as involved as possible in household tasks as well as personal and financial responsibilities. Just because a person has cancer and might need a great deal of rest does not mean that he cannot handle some tasks of day-to-day living. At the same time, family members need to be very sensitive to what the person is unable to do.

Dos and Don'ts for Caregivers Regarding Control

1. Don't assume that you are helping by taking control of decision making.
2. Don't treat the patient like a child, an invalid, or someone who is mentally incapacitated.
3. Don't take care of responsibilities that the patient is capable of handling.
4. Don't make decisions that the patient is capable of making.
5. Don't make assumptions about what the patient wants or needs; ask instead.
6. Do encourage the patient to be involved in decisions concerning his care and his life.
7. Do encourage the patient to handle whatever responsibilities she is able to.
8. Do respect the patient's choices.

9. Do try to be open with the patient.
10. Do be aware of the patient's need to be independent, capable, responsible, and needed.

Being a Listener

The stress of cancer makes communication in the family more difficult. One of the most helpful things family members can do is to allow and encourage the patient to talk about what he is feeling—and to listen. Such conversations, however, do not always come about naturally.

Family members often want to avoid conversations about the patient's emotional reactions. They might well find it painful and confusing to hear about the patient's feelings, particularly when they are trying to deal with their own. They might be alarmed and bewildered at the patient's fluctuating and intense emotional states, and try to avoid such communication to spare themselves hurt and feelings of helplessness. Some might even believe that it is not good for the patient to express negative feelings.

Patients also might tend to try to avoid such conversations. They might not want to upset their family members or perhaps they are not accustomed to expressing fear, anger, or sadness. (Men often find it hardest to acknowledge and express fear, while women often have a hard time with anger.) Dealing with their treatment, time lost from work, mounting financial pressures, and all the logistical difficulties involved in daily living, they might convince themselves that their emotions are less important than all their other challenges. Like family members, they might find it easier to show cheerfulness and optimism, rather than to let anyone see their fear, depression, and despair. Yet not being able to talk about what is most important and most troubling to them—their fears about their illness, pain, disfigurement, disability, and death—has several effects. Without being given expression, their fears increase, and they themselves remain isolated. Unless they can talk about what is paramount in their lives, they can become terribly lonely. When they can express these feelings, they feel less burdened by them: less depressed, less fatigued, and more energetic.

When the patient does express fears and concerns, however, family members might well cut off communication. They might change the subject. They might tell the patient not to worry, and to be positive because everything will turn out all right. They might feel the need to cheer the patient up, in part because they find the patient's emotions painful to hear.

> Tom expressed a very realistic fear when he said to his wife, Margaret, "I'm afraid about what is going to happen to you and Carl if I don't make it. He might not be able to finish college, and there's still a big mortgage on the house." Margaret responded, "Oh, don't think that way. You're going to be fine." Rather than acknowledging Tom's concerns, the effect of Margaret's denial was to invalidate them. It would have relieved Tom of these fears if he and Margaret had discussed them, considered their financial situation realistically, and begun some financial planning.

One of the greatest, most life-giving gifts family members can offer is to invite patients to talk about what is going on with them. One of the greatest gifts therapists can give family members is to try to teach them to accept the patient's feelings and to assure them that the best way to help is simply to listen. Many family members feel responsible for the patient's emotions and try to change them. Out of a misguided need to try to save the patient, they might try to cheer up or divert the patient when he is depressed. ("You look like you're feeling down. Let me tell you about a funny thing that happened today.") They might try to argue with the person's feelings. ("There's no reason to be afraid." "Don't cry." "You shouldn't be mad. That will only make you feel worse.") There is more to emotional support than offering hope and encouragement. People who are ill need to be heard and understood, not fixed, reassured, or soothed. They need their suffering understood and acknowledged. They need to be heard by someone who wants to listen and who understands.

Mara, recently diagnosed with ovarian cancer, said to her husband, Bob, "I'm terrified about what could happen. I'm so afraid I might die." Bob hugged her. "Yes, this whole situation has been very frightening." Encouraged, Mara went on to talk about her fears. She cried and talked about her anger at the unfairness of the illness as well. Bob held her hand and listened. When she relaxed, he said, "I know you're scared. I'm scared, too, because we don't know what's going to happen. But we'll keep doing everything we know to do to make you better."

Bob didn't argue with Mara's fears or try to deny or change them. He understood that her fears were real and important. He let her know with his words and his presence that he was there with her. After letting out what had been troubling her most, Mara felt better just having been heard and understood.

Acceptance of the patient's fears can be very important to the patient, but that acceptance should not be unconditional. Mara had real reason for her fears. However, when it is clear that a patient has mistaken ideas or is imagining the worst possible scenarios and then reacting as if they were true, those feelings can be questioned and challenged. ("I do understand that you're afraid, but your last test showed that the tumor is shrinking. That means the chemo is working. Don't you think that's true?" "Remember that the doctor explained that everyone reacts differently to the same drug, and that no one's reaction can be predicted. He said that some people have few reactions to that drug. You might be one of them.") Although family members themselves might also be susceptible to the same kind of thoughts that trouble the patient, they might be able to recognize and try to refute the patient's irrational beliefs.

Besides the patient's fears, family members might have to deal with the patient's irritability and anger. Patients may snap or lash out at apparently trivial problems. The patient might blame family members for incidents in the present or even for incidents in the past that were not discussed before. Particularly if the patient has not often acted angrily or assertively before, family members might be alarmed. ("She's never talked like that before.") The situation can be easier for them if they realize that the patient might be as alarmed as they are at her own uncharacteristic behavior, and even feel guilty about it afterward. Anyone undergoing cancer treatment is extremely sensitive, even hypersensitive, and likely to experience mood swings. It also helps if family members can remember to try not to take the patient's moods personally or to respond argumentatively. At the same time, there is no reason for them to accept harsh words from the patient. ("I know you're upset and angry, and feeling awful now. But you just hurt my feelings. It's not okay with me when you talk to me that way. Can we just discuss this?" "Let's stop this conversation. I don't want us to hurt each other or say things we don't really mean. Let's talk later when we're both not so upset.")

Although the patient might not openly express grief, it will be no secret to the family that the patient feels anguish at all the losses the illness has brought. It is not easy to hide. If it is apparent that the patient is trying to maintain a cheerful face (which, under the circumstances, has to be a false facade), the family can invite the patient to talk about what she is feeling. They can point out (as their psychotherapist might have pointed out to them) that crying is not a first step toward major depression. It does not result in depleting courage and strength, but does just the opposite by relieving tension and clearing the way for other feelings.

The patient might want to talk about the illness or not to talk about it. Both reactions are ways of trying to deal with the situation, and both need to be respected. The patient can be invited to talk about his feelings, without being pressured to do so. ("You look like something is bothering you right now. Do you want to talk about it?" "If there is ever anything on your mind that you want to talk about, I'm here.")

Just knowing that such an invitation is a standing offer and that it is genuine can be hugely supportive to the patient.

At times patients will welcome the company of family members and friends. At other times, for whatever reasons, they will want and need to be alone. The greatest help at such times is to respond to the patient's desire for companionship or allow him solitude.

Some Dos and Don'ts for Family Members Regarding Emotions

1. Don't argue with the patient's feelings.
2. Don't tell the patient what to feel.
3. Above all, don't tell the patient to think positively. This is guaranteed to make anyone who is ill feel worse by invalidating whatever natural reactions they might have.
4. Don't tell the patient what not to feel.
5. Don't try to fix or save the person. You won't succeed.
6. Don't deny or try to make light of their feelings and their suffering.
7. Don't be surprised at the patient's changed emotional state. Try not to take it personally.
8. Do remember that when the patient wants to talk, all you have to do is to listen silently.
9. Do understand that when the patient is talking, your silence is encouraging, for it means that you are listening. You might or might not understand the person's feelings, but there is no need to try to change them.
10. Do understand that sometimes the patient won't want to talk. Respect that need.
11. Do understand and accept that sometimes the patient needs to be alone. Respect that, too.
12. Do understand that anyone involved with cancer (including you, the family member) is likely to have mood swings, a progression of strong feelings that includes anger and irritability, fear and ter-

ror, sadness and grief, depression and hopelessness. It also includes love and hope.

13. Do understand that while you can be there in many ways, you cannot meet all the person's emotional needs. No one can.

Being a Cheerleader for the Future

If there is one most important way family members can help and support the patient, it is with their own conviction that the patient can get better. Their attitude about the patient's recovery is communicated in everything they do and say, and affects patients strongly. If their underlying feeling is despair, even though it is not expressed directly, the patient will find it difficult, if not impossible, to be hopeful. On the other hand, if family members convey hope, the patient can also believe in his own recovery.

Anyone dealing with cancer must learn to live with uncertainty. No one, not even the patient's physicians, can know what will happen. One of the most effective ways family members can help to lessen the patient's anxiety (as well as their own) and to encourage hope is to make plans for the future. Anyone with cancer can easily stop believing in their future. Planning the future is a way to help restore that belief. The family can discuss with the patient short-term wishes and long-term goals and dreams. Together they can figure out steps that can be taken, both now and later, to actualize them. By making plans based on his own authority rather than medical authority, the patient can move from feeling helpless to feeling empowered to act.

For example, a short-term goal might be a trip the patient has wanted to take. The family can schedule a date—for example, 2 months after the last chemotherapy treatment—and then arrange for tickets (along with travel insurance, just in case the plan goes awry). This not only gives everyone something exciting and vitalizing to anticipate, but also helps them believe that a future is possible and that they can shape it. Longer-term goals and dreams can also be discussed and planned, along with ideas about the steps that need to be taken to make them happen.

People with cancer often say that all they want is that their life be the same as it was before they were ill. However, that life is the context in which the cancer grew. The question now is, what does the patient really want to do in his life? What buried or deferred dreams does she have? What turns her on? Regardless of the patient's physical situation, the family can encourage and help her to begin planning and making changes so that her life can bring more enthusiasm and fulfillment. Clearly this has significant emotional effects. What is not as obvious is that it can also have significant physical effects.

From over 40 years of statistical and clinical research studies, psychologist Lawrence LeShan (1994), author of *Cancer as a Turning Point*, developed a psychotherapy approach for people with cancer. He found that when patients commit to finding and actualizing their own best and natural ways of being, relating, and creating that bring meaning and enthusiasm to their life, their health can improve. By making lifestyle changes and the psychological changes that lead them to do this, they appear to create an inner "healing climate" that increases their positive response to medical treatment (Bolletino, 2004).

From those studies, LeShan developed a new psychotherapy approach that he first used only with cancer patients. Unlike traditional medical and psychotherapeutic approaches based on the question, "What is wrong with you?" this therapy asks, "What is right with you?" "What kind of life would you find most meaningful and fulfilling?" and "What actions can you take and what changes can you make so that you move more in that direction?" Working toward creating a richer, more fulfilling life has resulted in survival time superior to that of traditional therapies focusing on psychological problems and past causes. When people with cancer make a commitment to finding ways to make their life more meaningful and fulfilling, this (theoretically) stimulates their self-healing abilities so that there is often a change in their body's ability to resist the cancer process.

Feelings and thoughts can neither cause nor cure cancer, but they are integral aspects of the whole person. As people make large or small changes in their lives that are significant to them, they are changing the ecology of their total being. They are changing the total environment in which the cancer grew. Although the approach was originally for cancer patients, it has been shown to be effective for others as well. Those who have recovered from cancer appear to increase their chances of nonrecurrence and those who are well, their chances of improving and maintaining their health.

Family members are not psychotherapists and cannot apply this psychotherapy approach and all that it involves. What they can do, however, is to encourage patients to begin thinking about how they can make their lives more fulfilling, and to take steps to begin moving in that direction. They are likely to find that patients are very receptive. One common effect of a cancer diagnosis is that it makes it very clear what is important and what is not. Patients, confronted with their mortality, often feel that they want to find out how to live more fully as who they are.

Chapter 8, which described the emotional world of people with cancer, included the story of Phil, the technical writer whose rage propelled him to lash out in all directions, notably toward other drivers on the road. As it turned out, that was only half the story.

Phil was my client. Sometimes his wife, Jenny, attended our weekly sessions. The first time we met, I explained to both of them about the kind of psychotherapy I do, and we discussed some simple things he might like to explore to enrich his life and to feel better. Within a few weeks he enrolled in a Saturday morning yoga class, began to exercise more, and consulted a nutritionist. He tried to spend more time with his teenage son Jon and to take Jenny out to dinner one evening a week.

Still, he often arrived at our sessions fuming about something or other, usually Washington politicians, world leaders, physicians, nurses, or commuters who drove too slowly. While his diatribes reflected his anger, sometimes they also revealed his sharp wit. One day, when he started to rant about the latest political news, I said, "Look, Phil. You like to write. You're articulate, and you have a lot to say. Why not write about your views, not just about politics but about all kinds of things—like your own experiences and how you feel about them? They might be in the form of a journal or some essays." He liked the idea of a different, more personal kind of writing, and said he would try it.

Two weeks later I was surprised to hear him say that he had set up a blog. In it, every stupidity and injustice in the world served as his target of the day. For the first time he sounded excited about something he was doing, and for the next month Phil's blog was his new vehicle for venting his rage. To be sure, writing a blog was far less dangerous than yelling while driving at 65 miles an hour, and his newborn enthusiasm was good to see. The problem was that instead of releasing his anger, his Internet tirades were fueling it.

Fortunately, he soon came to realize that himself. "The blog is going great, and I really get off on writing it. But you know? Whenever I read the paper or see the news, I get involved and angry, and when I get that angry my whole body gets tense and I get more tired. I think that maybe all this just isn't good for me. I think that maybe I should just stop doing the blog, and even stop trying to keep up with all the news."

"Yes! That's a very good idea. You like the writing part. So do you have any thoughts about what you might like to write instead?"

Phil smiled broadly. "As a matter of fact, I do. I have a great idea. I want to write some monologues on different subjects. Some will be funny. I really can be a funny guy, you know. I always had a secret wish to be a performer of some kind, maybe even a comedian, so my idea is that after I get enough monologues together, I'd like to perform them—in front of an audience."

Jenny, who was with him that session, said, "Phil told me about this last night. I think it's a wonderful idea." Turning to Phil, she said, "And you would be great at it. Besides, I'd rather be married to a comedian than a rabble-rouser."

So for the next 4 months, with whatever energy he had to spare, he worked on monologues. His weight loss began to be noticeable (although as a result, he looked more fit than before) and so were the darkening circles under his eyes. But Phil's mind and body were going in different directions. In important ways he was becoming more and more vitalized and alive. "I've rediscovered my love of writing," he said delightedly, "and I've been reading what I write to Jenny and Jon. So far they like it a lot." Occasionally he read a line or a few short passages to me. Some of his monologues were indeed funny, some were predictably bitter, some sharply insightful, some poignant. Together they covered the range of all that he had been feeling since he was diagnosed with cancer. Now that range had widened to include excitement, anticipation, and hope.

One session brought me to tears. It was the time he said he wanted me to hear an entire piece he had just completed, and to respond as if I were a critic. As I listened, it seemed clear that he had finally put into words the real ground of his rage. The monologue was about the injustice of having cancer.

When he felt he had nearly enough material, he found a drama coach and arranged for a few lessons to work on his delivery. He also booked a small hall with a stage to rent for an evening. Jon designed and printed announcements, and Jenny sent them out to friends and acquaintances 6 weeks in advance. (After much deliberation, Phil had decided that it would be all right to ask the people attending for a small admission fee, just enough to cover the cost of the hall.) Shortly before the performance, he and I spent a session discussing ways to deal with stage fright.

The performance was held during a week I had to be away. He told me afterward that he was delighted at how it went, that he had thoroughly enjoyed himself on stage, that more people than were expected had attended, and that he was surprised and gratified at the responses he received. ("They laughed in the right places, and some people were even crying," he marveled.) That initial success encouraged Phil to continue writing whenever he could. He continued to give private readings (in the bedroom) for his two most appreciative fans, Jenny and Jon. He put his essays up on a new blog, and from time to time performed some of them as monologues at a local comedy club.

The original prognosis that he had no more than a year to live was proven to be wrong. Although his cancer was an aggressive one, he responded far better to his treatment than his physicians had expected, and far outlived medical predictions.

During the last few months of his life he could no longer come to my office, so we spoke on the phone. One day when I called him turned out to be the day before he died. Jenny held the phone to his ear as I talked to him.

Several weeks later I received an envelope from Jenny. In a note she explained that she was enclosing the program from Phil's first stage performance with my name on it, which he had evidently forgotten to give me. On it he had written, "In the words of Yogi Berra, 'It ain't over 'til it's over.' Thanks with love, Phil."

The crisis of cancer changes everyone involved. It can bring them closer, prompt them to rearrange their priorities, and to live more fully. Family members can have an enormous influence on patients' responses to their illness and their life. Therapists can best support family caregivers by assuring them that even despite what might be a bleak medical prognosis, their emotional presence, their hope and encouragement can help their loved one get through the illness and help to bring their self-healing abilities to the aid of their medical treatment.

We cannot know what the future will bring. Joseph Campbell's words come to mind: "We must be willing to let go of the life we had planned so as to have the life that's waiting for us" (1991, p. 18).

CHAPTER 11

Children in the Family: Guidelines for Parents

A simple Child
That lightly draws its breath
And feels its life in every limb
What should it know of death?
Wordsworth, "We Are Seven"

Although family structures and situations vary widely, the changes and uncertainties that cancer brings invariably create fear and anxiety in members of every family. Cancer creates what has been aptly called *ambiguous losses* (Boss, 2000). Life goes on but is no longer familiar and predictable. Its customary patterns are lost. As family routines, roles, and responsibilities change, children might no longer receive the kind of time and attention they need and are accustomed to. The parent who is ill is there, but not there: physically present (at least part of the time), but not present in the ways that the child has known.

Steve normally spent long hours in his office. Now with late-stage cancer, he spent all his time at home and most of that time in bed.

He was able to do some work there on his computer, and friends and colleagues visited him in the bedroom. He could rarely have dinner with his family, and on most days his wife, Lynn, prepared and brought him special meals. On days that he felt well enough, he spent time in the afternoons with his children, Ricky, 7, and Elise, 9. As soon as the children got home from school, they came directly into the bedroom and talked to him about their day. Sometimes Steve was able to play board games with them or tell them stories. Although he saw the children far more during the week then he could before his illness, he could no longer go outside to play rough-and-tumble games with his little boy. One day Ricky whispered to the school bus driver, "I miss my daddy."

Children are forced to change their perceptions of the patient. Life, losing its regularity and clarity, becomes ambiguous and uncertain, and children no longer know what to expect.

Young children interpret everything important that happens in their family as being caused by them: by something they did or didn't do, or by who they are. They might believe that they caused the illness or contributed to it in some way, or that they can make it better or worse. (From there, if the parent dies, it is a very small step to the magical belief that they caused that, too.) The importance of dealing with such misconceptions as soon as possible cannot be overestimated—even if the child denies having the belief.

Greg had two surgeries, chemotherapy, and radiation. When he wasn't in the hospital, he was at home in bed, where friends and relatives visited, and where he tried to keep up with some work on the computer. When he was awake, his children sometimes lay down next to him. Greg and his wife noticed that their son Jonny, normally a bright, active 6-year-old, had begun to behave strangely. From time to time he pulled the sleeves of his sweater down below his fingers and ran around in circles flapping his hands and muttering, "Dumb Jonny."

Greg knew his son well and had a good idea about what was going on. After several such incidents, he called Jonny into the bedroom and patted the bed next to him. Jonny jumped up and sat down.

Greg said, "Jonny, if you could fix me, would you?"

The boy replied immediately, "Oh, yes, Daddy."

Greg then asked gravely, "And would you charge me a lot of money to do that?"

"Oh no, course not, Daddy."

"I know that, Jonny. You're a very, very good boy. But, you see, you can't fix me. You're just 6 years old. You don't have that kind of power. But someday you're going to grow up and then you'll be very strong and powerful." (At this point Greg pushed up the sleeves of his pajama top and raised his arms with elbows bent and fists up, in the position of a weight lifter flexing his muscles.) He continued, "And at that time you'll be able to help people in any ways you want to."

Jonny grinned, raised his arms, and made tight fists in imitation of his father's posture. Then he gave Greg a quick hug and ran out of the room.

That was the end of Jonny's strange behavior. Instead, from time to time the little boy stopped whatever he was doing, stood up very straight, smiled, pulled up his sleeves, and extended his arms at his sides with elbows bent and fists tight, just like a very large man who was very strong and powerful.

Besides having false ideas, it is almost inevitable that children are afraid that the parent will die, that something will also happen to the well parent, or that they themselves will be left with no one to take care of them. Even while adults themselves are trying to deal with what is happening, they need to help and reassure the children.

This chapter offers suggestions for parents in providing that help and reassurance. There are steps they can take to try to correct children's mistaken ideas, lessen their fears, and give them some reassurance, beginning when they first tell the child about the cancer diagnosis.

Talking About the Diagnosis

There is no question about whether or not to tell a child that a parent or other loved one has cancer. Sooner or later, children see that the parent is sick. They need to know what is happening (Simonton, 1989). The best thing parents can do for them is to tell them what is going on to the extent they can understand and handle the information. Besides, trying to keep the diagnosis a secret to protect a young child is a bad idea certain to backfire. It is impossible to keep such a secret. From what is happening around them, children know that something terrible is happening. Maybe for the first time they see a parent cry. Maybe a parent stops talking to them and goes into the bedroom to be alone. Maybe the adults around them seem tense, upset, and anxious, and have long hushed discussions. Maybe they leave without explaining where they are going or make phone calls at night. The child knows that something is terribly wrong, and feels frightened and helpless (Simonton, 1989).

Without explanations children are likely to feel anxious and excluded. They might conclude that whatever is going on is too terrible even to talk about, and then imagine the very worst. They might feel guilty, assuming that whatever is happening is because of something they said or did. They might conclude that certain subjects are not supposed to be talked about, and then bury their fears. Children have vivid imaginations, and what they might invent in their imagination can be far worse than the reality. If parents do not involve them, if they pay less attention to them, or if a parent is hospitalized, children can easily believe they are no longer loved (Heiney, Hermann, Bruss, & Fincannon, 2001).

The way children react to news about cancer in the family depends in large part on who tells them, when and how they are told, what they are told, and how the adults closest to them are reacting.

Who Should Tell

Children should be told about the diagnosis from the people closest to them: the nuclear family, along with any other relative or close family friend. It can be extremely reassuring if the patient can be involved to explain what is happening. If this is not possible, a teacher, minister, school psychologist, social worker, or nurse might be called on to help.

When to Tell

Before telling a child of the diagnosis, parents might decide to speak with the child's teachers or guidance counselor. Not all details need to be given, but only enough for them to understand the reason if the child begins acting differently or having problems, and to intervene appropriately.

The first discussion with the children should be planned shortly after the diagnosis and before treatment begins. Parents should deliver the news when there is likely to be plenty of uninterrupted time for explanations, questions, and discussion. They should keep in mind that depending on how the child reacts, it might be best to continue explanations at another time.

It is best to wait for a time when they are at home with the child and feel able to talk fairly calmly. This does not mean that they should plan to hide their emotions or pretend that nothing is wrong. Children can deal with some expression of emotions from their parents, but this needs to be controlled. Children's responses will be shaped in part by the emotions that the parents convey. The calmer the parents when they impart the news, the less frightened the children are likely to be—although in any case they are likely to respond with fear and tears.

How to Tell

Before telling children about the diagnosis, parents would do well to give some thought to what they want to say and how to say it. This depends, of course, on the age of the child. Accurate information needs to be conveyed in a way the child can comprehend, in clear language the child can understand. It needs to be explained in a way that does not make it sound too frightening. For this reason, when there is more than one child in the family it might be helpful to talk with each one individually, or to talk with all of them first and then each one alone.

During the explanation, parents should make sure that the child understands what has been said. The child might be asked to repeat the information. The parent might ask if there are any words she didn't understand, or if there is anything she wants to ask.

What to Tell

Information need not and should not include everything the parents know. Children need to know only how what is happening will affect their lives. In general, what they are told depends on their age, their personality, and what the parents know about the medical situation.

Parents might tell young children no more than that the patient is sick and then wait for them to ask questions before explaining more. If they ask questions, they are ready for more information. If they stiffen, pull back, or become angry or defensive, they are probably not ready to hear more. It will be clear from their reactions how much information they are ready to handle.

Whatever children are told, they will need to assimilate the information at their own pace. Depending on their reactions, it might be best to have more than one discussion to give them additional information at a later time. They need to be told enough so they know what is happening and what to expect so they can begin to prepare for the changes about to happen in their lives.

Depending on the child's age, the following facts need to be imparted in as many discussions as necessary and repeated as often as necessary.

The patient has cancer. ("We've learned that Daddy has cancer." "Grandpa is in the hospital because he has cancer.") To very young children, it might be better not to mention cancer at all. ("Mommy is sick.")

Cancer is an illness but it is not contagious. Children need to be reassured that neither the parent who is well nor the child himself will also get sick (Babcock, 1997). ("Cancer is a serious illness, but most people who have cancer get well again. It isn't like the flu or a cold. No one can catch it from someone who has it. [The well parent] is not going to get it and you aren't going to get it. We can still hug and kiss [the patient].")

The child did not cause the illness. ("No one knows what causes cancer, but we do know that no one can cause anyone else to get it. It can't happen because of anything you or anybody did. It isn't anybody's fault. Doing something bad, or saying or thinking something bad can't cause cancer and can't make it worse. Doing or saying or thinking something good doesn't make it better. Nothing [the patient] or any of us did or said has anything to do with the illness.")

The patient will be helped to get well. ("Daddy has very good doctors, and they are going to do everything they can to make him better. He is going to take all his medicine and do everything he can to get well.")

Talking About Immediate Changes

Children need to know what to expect: how they will be cared for if a parent is sick or hospitalized and what effects the illness will have on their lives.

1. Prepare the children for changes in their daily routine and rituals, explaining what will happen and who will be involved. ("On Tues-

day I'll go to the hospital for a few days so the doctors can take care of me and help me." "Starting tomorrow Daddy will be going to the doctor's office every day in the afternoons for a treatment, and I'll go with him. Grandma will be here with you every day while I'm gone.")

2. Reassure children that their daily activities and routines will not change. ("While we are at the doctor's office, Danny's mom will drive you to baseball practice. We'll be back in time for all of us to have dinner together.")

3. Reassure children that whatever is happening, they are loved and not forgotten. ("There might be times that I can't be with you, or times that I'm thinking about other things, but that doesn't mean that we don't love you all the time." "There will always be someone here to take care of you.")

4. Reassure the children that the present situation is temporary.

5. Always maintain and convey hope.

Talking about Treatment

Tell the children exactly what you intend to do by way of a game plan. Explain the treatment plans in positive terms, rather than emphasizing negative side effects. ("I'll be going for a treatment called radiation every morning for 6 weeks, and I'll be home when you come back from school. After Christmas, I'll start a different treatment.") To help them feel confident and positive, show them that you are (Girard, 2001).

Prepare the children for changes in the patient. ("The doctors will be giving me special medicine to make the cancer go away. At first, the medicine might make me feel bad." "Daddy's treatment will make him very tired. Sometimes he will want to stay in bed." "Daddy won't come down to eat with us every night because he has trouble eating." "Mommy will be getting a treatment called chemotherapy that will cause her to lose her hair. When the treatment is finished, her hair will grow back.")

Explain how long the treatment will last. ("Daddy's chemotherapy treatments will be over by Halloween, but he will probably still be tired for a while after that." "I'll be finished with my radiation treatments by the time school is over, and then I'll be home with you every day." "We're expecting that Mommy will be home from the hospital next week.")

Talking About Changes to Come

To minimize anxiety, bewilderment, and fear, children need to be prepared for the many changes about to happen in their lives.

Explain who will be responsible for maintaining household activities, such as cooking and taking children to various activities. ("While we go to the hospital every day for a while, Aunt Ann will be picking you up from school. We'll be back not long after you get home.")

Explain how roles will be changing, and discuss ways that children might help with household responsibilities. Discuss what tasks can be shared and how chores can be divided. Include the children by asking for their help and involve them in decisions about what they might do. Whenever possible, children should be given regular age-appropriate tasks so they feel they have some control by being able to do something. ("Mommy won't be able to do the things in the house she usually does, so we can help.") For older children, it might be necessary to set up extra responsibilities (making sandwiches for lunches, doing the dishes, helping with house cleaning, taking out the trash). Let them know that their help is welcome and let them choose their degree of involvement.

Answering the Dreaded Question

"Are you going to die?" is the question that all parents dread. It is also the one that children might be afraid to ask. Whether they ask or not, it needs to be addressed because it concerns the child's greatest fear.

There is no way for anyone to know whether someone with cancer will die of the illness. It depends on the response to treatment. Cancer is not usually a terminal illness, although it can be a chronic one. Uncertainty is one of the hardest things for everyone in the family to deal with.

If there is good reason to believe that the patient will recover, that is what the child should be told. ("Mommy should be fine after her treatment.") If the patient's prognosis is uncertain, parents can say that everything is being done to help the patient get well. ("We hope that Daddy will be all right. He and the doctors will be doing everything they can to make him better. He will be getting very good treatment that we hope will cure him." "Grandma is very sick. The doctors are working hard to make her better. We don't know what will happen and it's hard not to know, but we hope she will be all right again, and I know you hope so, too.")

Whatever the situation, be realistic and honest. If it is known that the patient has only a short time to live, do not give the children false reassurance by telling them that everything will be all right. With unrealistic expectations, they will have a far more difficult time when the patient dies. What is helpful is to prepare them for what is going to happen (Heiney et al., 2005).

Initial Reactions

There is no such thing as a normal reaction that can be expected. Different children react differently. The way they react is their way of handling the news. Some children react with denial, some with anger or tears, some with calmness, and some with concern for others in the family. They might express one feeling at first and a different one later. What they need most is that their parents understand and accept whatever they feel.

Parents are well advised to encourage children to express their emotional reactions. Explain that when someone has cancer, it is natural for the people who love them to feel surprised, sad, angry, and frightened. ("I know it's hard for you to believe that Mommy is sick. She doesn't feel sick. But it's true. The doctor told us that she has cancer, and we're upset about it, too." "It's okay to cry. Daddy's illness makes me very sad. Sometimes I cry. You might feel sad, too." "Sometimes I feel angry because Mom is sick. You might feel angry sometimes, too." "It's awful that Dad is ill. I know how scared you must be. I want you to know that you will never be alone. We all love you, and someone will always take care of you.")

It is very reassuring to a child for parents to demonstrate that they are not afraid of the child's feelings and want only to be supportive and understanding.

At times it can also be helpful to try to channel the child's feelings. ("I'm frustrated [or sad or angry], too. Why don't we go outside together and take a walk?") Later, the parent might ask the child to talk about her feelings. If the child is old enough, the parent might ask her to write down the way she feels, and add that when she has done this, the parent will look at what she has written. If the child draws pictures, ask what he has drawn, but do not try to interpret what the child draws or says about the drawing.

Ways to Help the Child

Regardless of the children's ages, they will need individual help and support to work through the complex situation that cancer brings. Below are some guidelines to help them (Babcock, 1997; E. LeShan, 1986; Pomeroy, 1996).

1. Continue to be honest with the children. Explain what is happening in terms they can understand, always balancing truth with re-

assurance and hopefulness. Assure them that they will continue to be told what is happening.

2. Answer questions honestly. If you are not open with children, they might not ask questions. Do not leave them to imagine what is happening, for what they imagine will invariably be far worse than the reality. If you don't know the answers, say that you will try to find out.

3. To whatever extent possible, try to maintain normalcy by minimizing changes in the children's daily life. To feel secure and to know that their entire world has not been disrupted, children need their regular routines and schedules (mealtimes, storytime, playtime, bedtime). Encourage them to continue all their usual activities (Fitzgerald, 1999; Heiney et al., 2001). If the patient is going far away for treatment, leave children at home, except for short visits. They can maintain connection with the patient by making phone calls, or sending letters, photographs, or tapes of their activities. Uprooting children usually requires them to make too great an adjustment and deprives them of their home, their normal activities, and their friends.

4. Allow and ask for help from others. Trying to keeping children's lives as much the same as possible is not easy when parents are involved in patient care, medical appointments, or trips to the hospital. This is a time to accept help from others—for example, by preparing dinner for the family, driving a child to an activity, staying with a child during times of active medical treatment, or staying with the patient while a parent attends a child's function. This is a time that children need extra care, attention, and support from parents, other close relatives, and friends.

5. Encourage children to help in any ways that are appropriate. Having them do something for the patient or the household is an effective antidote to worrying and feeling helpless.

6. Continue to maintain and enforce the same rules, boundaries, and discipline consistently, with the same degree of firmness or flexibility as before. Even if it is obvious that the child is acting up to

get needed attention, discipline is at least as necessary as it always has been. In times of upheaval in family life, controls are often put aside. This can create anxiety in children, for it clearly communicates that something is very wrong. In times of stress, they are not ready to make choices, and they need to know that their parents are still in control. To the greatest extent possible, household rules, limits, and discipline all need to remain in place. Setting limits and maintaining them is especially important for older children whose misbehavior can have serious, even disastrous, consequences.

7. Make time for fun by creating good times as often as possible. Acknowledge and celebrate children's scholastic or athletic achievements, holidays, birthdays, and family milestones. Create special occasions, such as outings for the children or simple "coming home from the hospital" celebrations for the patient. Rent videos of funny movies so the family can laugh together. (Any time spent laughing is good for everyone in the family.) Take the children to the zoo, an early movie, or a museum. Cancer is a part of their life, but don't let it become all of it.

8. Try not to let the children see the patient in pain. If the patient is in the hospital, arrange visits with the children at a time the patient is comfortable. If the patient is at home, arrange with the doctors for pain control.

9. Involve the children in every possible way so that they feel included, wanted, and needed. Do not encourage them to ignore or avoid what is a real part of their lives. All the children in the family can take on age-appropriate household tasks in ways that they choose. Young children can help the patient by bringing things to her or reading aloud. Older children can participate in family discussions. The family can meet together regularly to discuss everything going on in the family (not just cancer), and to plan ways to deal with changes in family routines.

10. Offer choices so that children can have some sense of control. ("Would you rather stay here with Dad or come with me to the grocery store?" "We'll all need to help while Mom isn't feeling

well. Would you like to set the table or take out the trash?" "I'm going to rake some leaves in the yard. Would you like to help with that?")

11. Encourage children to express their thoughts and feelings, and also let them know that sometimes it's okay if they don't want to talk.

12. Let the children know every day that they are important. When parents are preoccupied with other concerns and don't give children the time and attention they usually get, they can easily feel hurt, neglected, or unloved. Let them know every day that they are loved.

13. Let the children be children. While it helps them to take on some responsibilities, do not allow them to become adults by becoming caregivers to younger children or confidants of a parent.

Later Reactions

Clearly children's reactions depend on the entire situation. A parent's illness is more difficult for them if the treatment continues for a long time. As treatment goes on, the patient is likely to be feeling sick and unable to continue the usual responsibilities. The other parent might be exhausted and unable to be as attentive as usual to the children's needs, or to be with them in ways they have come to expect (Heiney et al., 2001). The situation is also more difficult if the parents are not getting along, or if they are divorced or separated. If there has been illness or death in the family before, the children's reactions will be strongly influenced by that experience. Whatever the situation, they are certain to be distressed.

It can be extremely helpful if therapists prepare their clients for reactions they might observe in their children, and alert them to those for which they might want to seek help. For example, children might show their fears and anxiety by becoming depressed and withdrawn. They might try to avoid what is happening by distracting themselves with television or by spending more time away from home. They might have dreams that frighten them. They might act up or regress in some ways—for example, by becoming upset at any brief separation from a parent or by misbehaving to get the attention they need. They might become agitated or hostile. There might be changes in their eating or sleeping. They might begin to have physical complaints, such as headaches or stomachaches. They might have difficulty concentrating, and their school grades might suffer. They might distance themselves from the person who is ill because they don't want to burden the patient, or because they don't know how to deal with the patient's changed appearance or behavior.

They might become angry—at the cancer, at the patient for being ill, at all the changes in their lives, or at having to do things that their parents normally did. They might be angry at getting less attention, or at being unable to do some of the things they usually do. They might be angry simply because their life has suddenly changed in unexpected ways. They might be angry because they are frightened. (It is far easier to feel anger than to face underlying fear.) What children need is for their feelings to be acknowledged and understood. ("You're angry, and I wonder if you're mad because Mom is sick.") It is very helpful for parents to demonstrate that they are not afraid of the child's feelings and want only to be supportive and understanding. Along with that acknowledgment, it is important that adults set limits, if necessary. ("You're mad, but it's not okay to throw things, or to yell. It's never okay to hurt the cat.") Make the children's reactions a topic to be discussed with them.

If families follow the suggestions in this chapter, usually children's disturbed reactions do not last long. If they persist and a child continues to be depressed, withdrawn, or angry for several weeks or longer, parents would do well to seek professional help. They can speak with the child's teachers or school counselors, or consult therapists or counselors who specialize in working with young children (Alpha Institute, 1998).

Any child whose parent has been diagnosed with cancer needs help and support. There are programs that support younger children and teenagers in person or online.

In summary, when a parent has cancer, the children's most important needs are (Seligman, 1996):

1. Clear information and ongoing communication that balances honesty with hopefulness;
2. Reassurance that the child had nothing to do with the patient's illness;
3. Reassurance that there will always be someone to take care of them;
4. Reassurance (with words, actions, and physical affection) that they are involved, important, and loved;
5. Encouragement and opportunities to express feelings and thoughts;
6. Maintenance of normal routines and activities; and
7. Maintenance of normal rules and discipline.

People find their own ways to cope with cancer, and each family needs to discover what works best for them. Parents' emotional openness gives children tacit permission to express their own feelings. Parents' honesty about what is happening gives the children permission to ask questions and minimizes their anxieties and fears. Parents' openness with their children during the crisis of cancer sets the foundation for the child's trust in them and shapes their relationship with them during the illness and in the future.

The way adults in the family cope with the crisis of cancer and all the day-to-day difficulties it brings teaches their children that people can carry on and do their best even in extremely challenging circumstances.

CHAPTER 12

Dealing With Recurrence

Once more unto the breach, dear friends, once more
Shakespeare, *Henry V*, III, i, 1

For most people who have had cancer, the end of medical treatment is not the end of fear. After treatment ends, usually their greatest source of anxiety is the possibility of being diagnosed again. For months, even years afterward, at the slightest pain or discomfort anywhere in their body, they conclude that cancer is back. They fear that some cancer cells were not destroyed and will spread, or that a different cancer will appear. In time such fears recede, but they do not disappear, for they are not wholly unwarranted. Recurrences happen. Months or years following treatment, some former patients are diagnosed again with an active cancer.

They and their families are often more upset at a recurrence than they were at the original diagnosis. They are likely to react initially with the same shock, disbelief, fear, grief, anxiety, and depression that they felt the first time. This time, however, they might feel more helpless, more pessimistic, and more hopeless.

Patients might have a greater sense than before of a loss of control. ("I did everything I could. I suffered through all that. I did all the right things, and nothing worked.") They might be more depressed than after their initial diagnosis. Often they are angry again, but this time also at the medical team and at the treatments that failed them. They might have a loss of faith, believing they will not recover no matter what they do. They might blame themselves for having acted in ways that might have caused their recurrence, and doubt themselves for having made what now seems to have been the wrong medical choices. They might feel that they can't face the prospect of more surgery or chemotherapy. ("I just can't do this again, and anyway there's no point in trying.") Discouraged after their initial treatments did not work, some patients are unwilling to go back to the drawing board to learn about their present medical options and go through treatment again. ("I did everything I could the first time. Why should I do it again?") Some reject conventional medical options altogether, and opt for less punishing alternative treatments even though they might be unproven. Some might cling to the belief that prayer or determination alone will cure them.

Family members might well feel drained emotionally and financially. Like the patient, they might be frightened, depressed, discouraged, pessimistic, and even hopeless. They, too, might be angry at the doctors for not bringing about a lasting cure. Their anger might be directed at the patient for causing them more grief, and they might resent or blame the patient for having cancer again. They might blame themselves as well for having failed in some way. Like the patient, they might feel discouraged and overwhelmed at the prospect of another upheaval in their lives after all their efforts and hard work. ("I thought it was all over. I can't go through all that again.") The idea of more patient care, further financial outflow, more time away from work, and the need to ask relatives and friends for help and support again might be more than they feel they can handle. A wife might be more threatened than before at the loss of security. A husband who is less accustomed to concerning himself with meals and children's activities might feel more resentful than before. At the same time, family members are likely to be even more afraid than before that the patient might die. Their emotional stress is likely to be compounded by their unwillingness to communicate their thoughts and feelings to the person who is ill again.

Psychotherapy for family members involved with recurrence is in many ways the same as for an initial diagnosis. All their reactions need to be expressed, clarified, and sorted out; only in this way can they be managed and lessened. Now, however, if the patient and family have not at least begun to look into medical treatment, the therapist needs to determine the emotional reactions blocking them from doing so. Some patients and families, so discouraged by the reappearance of cancer, give up or opt for questionable alternative treatments without first determining whether conventional treatments are likely to be effective.

Also, if family members have not yet talked about their fears and anxieties that this time the patient will die, this is surely the time to do so. Again, as with an initial diagnosis, clients need to understand that whatever they feel is all right and to accept their emotions. There are no "shoulds" or right and wrong when it comes to feelings.

Besides clarifying and validating clients' emotional reactions, another task of the therapist after a rediagnosis is to provide accurate information. Many people, including those with cancer and their family members, have a mistaken idea about cancer and recurrence. They believe that the course of cancer is either straight up (the patient is treated, recovers, and remains cancer free) or straight down (the patient is treated, the treatment doesn't work and cancer returns or spreads, and the person dies). Clients need to be told that while both of these scenarios can happen, they are not the only possibilities (Simonton, 1989). The therapist can allay their fears and help them make sound decisions and realistic plans.

The therapist can make it clear that recurrence does not always mean death. There are effective medical treatments for recurrent and metastatic cancers.

Some patients undergo treatment for a recurrence and then remain cancer free.

Some have recurring cancers that grow so slowly that there are no symptoms, and physicians might decide not to treat them for years.

Some patients have more than one recurrence and undergo treatment each time. For them cancer becomes a chronic illness. In this situation the medical aim is not to cure but to control the cancer—hopefully until a cure is found. Many kinds of recurring cancers are controlled for years by surgery, radiation, chemotherapy, or hormonal therapies. Many patients with more than one recurrence live longer today than ever before (Holland & Lewis, 2001).

The All-Important Choice

After an initial period of shock, grief, anger, and despair when they are diagnosed again, some patients have no doubt that they want to do everything to get well, no matter what it takes. With their families they take action as before, consulting physicians and making treatment decisions and plans. Some patients are reluctant to go ahead with treatment, but because they want to live, they do so. For others, however, their first reactions do not abate. They assume that further treatments will be useless, and they become depressed and passive.

In this case, although family members might also be discouraged, they can best help by informing the person who is ill that there is a choice to be made. They can ask the all-important question, "Do you want to make a new commitment to working toward getting well, or do you want to die? We love you very much. If you weren't with us, we would miss you terribly, but we will support you in whatever you decide." That choice is solely the patient's (Simonton, 1989).

It is of no help for family members to intervene with their own opinions, making such comments as, "Don't even think about dying. Everything will be fine," or, on the other side of the coin, "Maybe you should just face the fact that you're not going to get well." Instead, along with expressing their love, they can best help by making it very clear that the patient must make the decision, and that they respect the patient's autonomy. (It needs to be noted here that if the family member learns that the patient has decided to give up, even though medical treatment might help, supporting that decision can be extremely difficult for therapists.)

The cancer patient might need time. For some people the choice is not an easy one. Even if they decide to go for life, they know that the outcome will be uncertain. No one can know how successful renewed medical treatment would be, and treatment involves more burdens on the family. What is most important, however, is that patients be aware that it is a choice, and that the choice is theirs. They might want to look carefully into all their options. They might express the wish to talk to a doctor about whether dying would be painful, or to talk to a clergyman about death. If the patient seriously considers the possibility of dying, this does not mean that he has given up on living, but only that he is taking the choice very seriously (Simonton, 1989). Very often someone who considers death carefully is very likely to do everything possible to live.

John had late-stage cancer that had spread and could not be cured. All his physicians could do was to keep him pain free and comfortable. He had an old friend, Dave, who was a doctor. John spoke with Dave and explained how important it was for him to have choices about his life when his range of choice had been diminishing steadily. He told Dave how demoralizing and depressing it was to feel increasingly helpless. At the end of their discussion, Dave agreed to give him some pills that he could take if he decided to end his life. John hid the pills away. Simply knowing that he had them gave him a sense of control that made all the difference to his desire to live. He never took the pills, and later died in the hospital.

Faced with a rediagnosis, patients and families often forget that they have some things going for them that they didn't have the first time:

- They know more about cancer and treatments than they did after the initial diagnosis.
- They know more about medical resources and have established relationships with doctors and hospitals or treatment centers.
- They have already set up sources of support.
- They have already developed coping strategies.

They also need to be reminded that there are effective medical treatments for recurrent cancer. If there are no viable medical options, there might be non-conventional treatments that can help. In many situations some alternative treatments have prolonged some patients' lives and even brought about recoveries. Despite the attitude of many physicians, choosing alternative treatments does not mean choosing a hopeless cause. If conventional medical treatment is unlikely to help or if the patient rejects it, family members should be encouraged to investigate alternative treatments to determine if any of them seem right for the patient.

Besides providing such information, another of the therapist's tasks is to help family members cope with their situation. This includes helping them to develop realistic hopes and build confidence in their ability to make plans and sound decisions (Seligman, 1996). Negative thinking is not the only alternative to positive thinking. The alternative to both is realistic thinking: having the courage to take steps to prepare for whatever happens.

It is never the case that nothing more can be done. There is always something, if not to increase the duration of life, then at least to improve its quality. There are many cases in which alternative treatments have done both.

CHAPTER 13

When the Patient Is Dying

It was beginning winter,
An in-between time . . .
Theodore Roethke, "The Lost Son" (1948)

For some patients medical treatment does not bring about a cure.

The patient's oncologist might say that aggressive treatment is no longer the right approach. Some patients might decide themselves that they cannot tolerate further toxic and costly treatments. Others, hoping to extend their lives even for a short time, choose to continue with them. They might be unwilling or unable to acknowledge that nothing can save them and want aggressive treatment for whatever extra time it can bring. Some are reluctant to stop treatment because they are afraid of being cut off from care, and then dying. They might fear (with some justification) that if they stop treatment, their doctor will abandon them. Sometimes it is the doctors who do not acknowledge that further aggressive treatment cannot help (and can only harm) or fear that stopping treatment will destroy the patient's hopes (Brody, 2008).

If the cancer is incurable, sooner or later, at some point, the goal needs to change to palliative treatment intended to keep the patient comfortable.

When the patient is dying, those closest to him feel that they are dying too. Most people with an incurable cancer do not die suddenly. Their death is preceded by a long period in which they and their families go through a physical and emotional struggle in which the forces of life and death contend. During that time they might find treatments and resources that can extend the patient's life. The patient and family should be reassured that the future is indefinite. Life should continue to be led with the understanding that no one can know when it will end. To be sure, there might well be better days and worse days, but to focus on death too early deprives everyone in the family of life that is still happening.

As the cancer progresses, demands on family caregivers increase after they have already provided months or even years of care. The stress on them of the ongoing illness and disability is enormous and becomes more intense as the patient comes closer to death. Because the patient now has needs around the clock, family caregivers shoulder more tasks and responsibilities than before. They might feel physically, emotionally, and financially drained as never before. As the patient experiences more severe symptoms, becomes increasingly dependent, and is slipping away from life, family caregivers, already in a fragile and vulnerable state, might be required to expend even more physical exertion and emotional endurance. Some push themselves to take on more than they reasonably can. At the same time as they watch helplessly as the patient suffers, they must make critical decisions about end-of-life treatment and care.

We live in a culture that has often been described as death denying and death defying. We regard the possibility of our death as remote from us and retreat from its reality. At the same time, we feel anxious about our mortality and that of those close to us. This makes it more difficult to deal honestly and openly with the reality (Jackson, 1983). Like most people in our culture, the average family members retreat from the reality of death. If they recognize the outcome of the patient's illness, they usually try to deny it, if not to themselves then to the patient. Death is kept out of their conversation. They want to protect themselves and might believe they are protecting the patient. Communication within the family often becomes strained as the family's attempts at cheerfulness become artificial and hollow. Although family members are likely to be more depressed and angrier than before, they try to protect the patient from undue stress. They often hide their feelings, put on a smiling mask, and try to reassure themselves as they reassure the patient. ("Everything will work out and you'll be all right. Just keep fighting. You have good doctors, and you're getting the best treatment.") In effect they are saying, "We won't let death in to get us." If the dying person tries to bring up the subject, family members turn them off. ("Don't talk like that. You're going to be fine.") Deception surrounds the entire family. Everyone, usually including the patient, pretends not to know. Family members do not realize that their genuine emotions would be much easier for the patient than their false smiles, which the patient doesn't believe anyway. As long as they all maintain their hollow reassurances and pretense, their loneliness cannot be underestimated. At the time when, more than anything else, they need one another, they become increasingly isolated. Tolstoy described this situation vividly in *The Death of Ivan Ilyich*, his short novel about a man with cancer who is dying: "What tormented Ivan Ilyich most was the deception—their not wishing to admit what they all knew and what he knew, but wanting to lie to him, and forcing him to participate in that lie. . . . And he had thus to live all alone on the brink of that abyss with no one who understood or pitied him."

Sooner or later family members are forced to relinquish their illusion. It becomes more and more difficult to maintain it when their daily involvement with the dying patient underscores their helplessness against death. The patient usually knows already that he has a short time to live but doesn't want to tell the family. Eventually, however, a time comes when they must face the reality that the patient will not recover. Whoever is told by physicians how serious the illness is must decide what to say to the patient, other family members, and, most difficult and most agonizing of all, the children.

Whatever the family members' feelings about the patient, whatever their relationship has been, they are going through their own kind of death process. They are about to lose someone who has been an integral part of their life. Each day is colored with the knowledge of the inevitable separation and with the emotions this knowledge brings. When denial and pretense are forced to end and the family begins to speak more honestly, their loneliness eases. Sometimes at such moments they can become aware of the depth of their love for one another.

However, whatever has been involved in their relationships in the past will still be there when the patient is dying. If family members did not relate to one another deeply or lovingly before, they are unlikely to do so now. With more open communication, however, they might be able to express some deep feelings and resolve some problems. The impending death forces families to come together, sometimes in mutual support, sometimes to reopen old conflicts and wounds, sometimes to try to heal them (Zuckerman, 2000). Knowing that the patient is going to die often intensifies relationships. The family often cares more deeply and becomes more conscious of the patient's every need. (Sometimes, to be sure, family members become particularly attentive to the patient as a penance. They might feel guilt because they themselves are well when their loved one is so sick, or because their love is mixed with old, unresolved resentments.) Whatever the situation, when genuine communication can begin the family can be in closer relationship with the patient during the last days of his life. In so doing, they ease the patient's emotional pain—and their own.

That their relationships become closer and intensify can be destabilizing for family members. Their fear of the patient's death might keep them conflicted between wanting to be close and wanting to run away. A widow, describing her feelings when her husband was dying, wrote, "It's a tug of war sometimes. How do you remain in a relationship with a dying person and also prepare yourself for his death, which is going to mean some distancing?" (Caine, 1990, p. 27). Each person needs to find her own answer to this. Family members closest to the patient sometimes withdraw their emotions because they are so afraid. In this situation, the therapist needs to point out that the pain of withdrawing might well be far greater than the pain of their later loss.

If family members can communicate openly and discuss their fears and concerns, they will be better able to make important decisions sooner, when there is more time and less pressure. As the cancer progresses and the patient become more dependent and debilitated, decisions need to be made about treatment and care, management of family responsibilities, and legal and financial matters. If these issues are raised in therapy, the therapist can help the family member to clarify and consider their choices so that they and the person who is ill can make decisions and take actions that are best for them.

Ways the Therapist Can Help the Family Member

The therapist can provide information and options, explore and clarify the client's feelings and beliefs, and encourage closeness in the family.

Providing Information and Options

It is often necessary for families to decide where the patient should be cared for. Many people envision the ideal way to die as being at home, with relatively little pain and few complaints, in control of whatever they are still able to control, surrounded by people they love. Very frequently, however, because of physical and medical complications, the last stages of cancer can be too exhausting for both the patient and the family. The family might not be able to provide the care at home that is needed. At the same time they might dread the prospect of sending the patient to an institution to die. Hospice care by trained professionals is an option that patients and family members need to know about.

Hospices provide teams of doctors, nurses, counselors, and trained volunteers to address the medical, social, psychological, and spiritual needs of patients and families. Often family members are not aware that hospice care might be provided at home, as well as in hospitals or nursing homes. In the past, medical care, which might include pain management and oxygen, was for the sole purpose of keeping the patient comfortable. Patients were admitted for hospice care only if they stopped receiving medical treatment. For that reason, many patients rejected hospice services in favor of medical treatments that might prolong their lives. However, with advances in medicine that can even help patients with late-stage cancer, this either-or approach is no longer valid. A growing number of hospice programs, as well as insurers, have come to recognize the need for appropriate, even advanced, medical treatment for patients in hospice care.

Hospice workers provide such services as occupational therapy, nutritional information, and religious or secular counseling. It is noteworthy that some patients who choose hospice care over aggressive treatments often live longer and with less discomfort, because the toxic effects of chemotherapy can hasten death (Brody, 2008).

When family members are caring for the patient at home, another option they might not know about has to do with pain control. Watching someone die takes an emotional toll, and family members feel themselves to be victims of their helplessness. When the patient suffers uncontrolled pain, or physical or psychological distress, the family's suffering increases, too. They might even feel guilty at not being able to help the patient. Often they are not aware that the patient's symptoms usually can be managed. Eliminating pain may not be possible, but there are usually ways to reduce it. A physician might provide medications that can relieve physical and psychological pain. The patient's depression, anxiety, panic attacks, and sleeplessness are often the result of physical pain. There are medications that might relieve these symptoms without causing drowsiness. When the pain is relieved, the patient might be back, in contact with the family, and able to deal with life again. Besides medication, music, meditation, massage, guided imagery, hypnosis, and visits from family, friends, or clergy might also help to lessen the patient's physical or psychological pain. (Some complementary treatments that can ease pain are listed in Appendix 5.)

Once such pressing decisions have been made, these caregivers' greatest needs in therapy are to work through their own tangled emotions, to help the person who is dying, to find meaning in what is happening, and to arrive at some sense of completion.

Working Through Emotions

Whatever the client's feelings are, they need to be validated by the therapist and accepted by the client herself. At this time more than ever, family members need their therapist to care about them, to listen, and to get to know them more deeply. In their situation the chances are that there are not many people to whom they can talk freely about what they feel or believe. Getting their emotions out in the presence of someone who understands can be enormously healing. With the therapist's support, these clients can work through and resolve their feelings, whatever they might be.

In the process of discussing the client's emotions, it might come out that she is responding to previous experiences with loss and death that color her reactions to the present situation. Exploring such past losses to clarify their effects on the client now can be extremely helpful.

For the therapist to try to cheer up the client at this time is no more productive than family members' attempts to do so. Although false cheer can only ring hollow, a light touch of humor is almost always appreciated. Even in pain people can laugh, and it is good for family members to laugh at times they believe they are unable to.

When the patient is dying, family members are likely to go through all the emotions again that Elisabeth Kübler-Ross has described so vividly, plus some others. Besides denial, there is anger, guilt, depression, bargaining, sadness, and grief. Acceptance might be the hardest.

No matter how well the family understands that the patient's illness will not be cured, no matter how much knowledge they allow in, it is often impossible to take in the reality that the patient is actually going to die. Sometimes when family members first learn that the illness cannot be cured, their denial causes them to shop around from doctor to doctor, sometimes traveling to remote treatment centers, alternative practitioners, even psychics, in hopes of hearing someone say that it isn't true that the patient has to die. Their anger and resentment now might be directed at the medical team that failed to bring about a cure, at the hospital staff who have not provided perfect care, or at the physician who gave them the news. To whatever extent they take in the reality of the impending outcome, they feel grief at their loss to come.

They might blame themselves for not having done more or loved more, and want to do everything possible to try to make up now for missed opportunities. It usually does no good for the therapist to try to assure them that they have no reason to blame themselves. What is far more productive is to listen very carefully. It sometimes turns out that there is a much deeper reason for their guilt (Kübler-Ross & Kessler, 2005). Uncovering and airing such feelings can lessen the emotional burden on the client now. As the patient's death approaches, the client might be caught up in conflicting emotions, including irrational guilt for being well or longtime resentment at the person for something that happened years before.

Clients might feel that they are living in a limbo of excruciating loss and uncertainty as their lives are slowly headed nowhere. The more these clients can express, explore, and clarify their emotions before their loved one dies, the better able they will be to be present with the dying patient, and the less unbearable their loss will be for them later. Acceptance of the patient's impending death does not mean consent or agreement with it. It is simply the recognition that nothing can be done to change what is going to happen.

Listening

We therapists cannot rescue our clients from their situations, their loss, or their pain. Assuring them that their feelings are normal, for example, is useful information but cannot take away the feelings. All we can do is to try to lessen their suffering by our attentive and caring presence. Our clients know that we cannot fix their situation. They want us only to hear them and understand. It is often a rare experience for them to discover that whatever they say is listened to, and whatever they feel is accepted.

Clarifying Beliefs

Clients dealing with an impending death might well ask unanswerable questions. ("Why has this happened?" "Why has God done this to us?" "Do you believe that there is something else after we die?") The only honest answer to such questions is that while we might have an answer for ourselves, we have no answers for them. ("This is a question that human beings have always struggled with. There is no one right answer for everyone. Neither I nor anyone else is living in your situation. It is your thoughts and your feelings about this question that are important. What is your answer to that question?")

It is as completely misguided as it is unethical for therapists to espouse religious or spiritual convictions with clients. (The obvious exception is when clients come to us because of a religious or spiritual view they know we share.) When their loved one is dying, they are particularly open and vulnerable, too likely to accept without question anything we might say. If they accept our beliefs, that does not make those beliefs right for them. Neither does it make it right for therapists to misuse our authority in that way. If clients raise such religious or spiritual questions, we can best help by encouraging them to explore what they themselves believe. ("I think that you already have the answers you are looking for. What do you believe happens to us after we die?" "Have your beliefs changed in any way since Joe was diagnosed?")

There is an important exception to this. I do not hesitate to tell my clients my conviction that life has meaning, even if we don't always recognize immediately what it is. Then I might ask if they think there is meaning in what is happening in their lives now. In many of his works, Viktor Frankl makes the point that therapists must be committed to a faith in meaning in order to communicate it. Others have made the same point. "The professional has become so accustomed to keeping his feelings and convictions out of sight that he tends to deny the patient what they need, the feeling of assurance that comes from a person of faith. The therapist might have to communicate his own faith in meaning in order for the client to understand it" (Bowers, Jackson, Knight, & LeShan, 1964, p. 24).

Encouraging Closeness

The therapist can encourage clients to share their feelings with the patient while it is still possible to do so. In *Being a Widow*, Lynn Caine eloquently explains the importance of this:

> I had watched [my husband] deteriorate until he became someone I hardly recognized, and still I pretended he wasn't going to die. . . . We never shared our feelings, our fears, or our love in any way that connected us to the reality of his prognosis. The truth was that we were afraid to face it and too uninformed to know how damaging that was. . . . We should have wept and talked together about death, but I smiled, was cheerful, and talked of getting well, even though I knew it was a lost war. (1990, p. 19)

Finishing Unfinished Business

The therapist can ask what unfinished concerns or unresolved conflicts the client has and whether it would help to discuss them with the patient while it is still possible to do so. The therapist might explore what the client might wish to do or say to the patient or other family members while the patient is still living to restore closeness and bring completion to these relationships.

Helping to bring about closeness and completion before the patient dies is a great gift the therapist can give to the entire family.

Ways Family Members Can Help the Patient

Family caregivers are usually frustrated at their inability to take away the patient's illness and suffering, particularly when it becomes clear that the patient is unlikely to survive. The therapist can point out that, while caregivers cannot stop of the course of the illness, there are significant ways they can help to ease the time of dying.

The Emotional World of the Person Who Is Dying

Patients' reactions to the prospect of their death vary widely. This is true even of the same patient at different times. Some people reach the stage of physical and emotional exhaustion so that they no longer strive for life. Death then becomes a surcease. Some people appear to be unafraid of death and contemplate it with serenity, curiosity, or relief. Others, feeling cheated out of their future, go through many of the same deep and painful emotions as when they were diagnosed—but now even more intensely.

No matter how long a road some patients have traveled through ineffective treatments, they might not believe that their illness will not be conquered. Denial can take many forms. Some people simply deny their prognosis and refuse further medical treatment that might help to prolong their lives. In desperation to live longer, some choose to go on with costly, toxic medical treatments when there is little reason to believe they will help. Some shop around for more doctors and more examinations, hoping for a different report. Some cooperate with their doctors fully, and might even make funeral arrangements, but inwardly do not believe that their life is ending. Denial comes and goes. Few of us can contemplate the prospect of our own deaths. (It has been said that there are two things you cannot stare at steadily: the sun and death.) Even patients who are seriously ill may think about their own deaths for a while, and then have to turn their attention away in order to pursue life (Kübler-Ross, 1969). Whatever its manifestation, denial is a helpful and necessary reaction, allowing us to filter in the truth and take it in as we can handle it. Some people, unable to tolerate the idea of their own end, die in denial because it is their only way of coping. Family members can help the patient by accepting what he feels, without arguing or contradicting him to try to break down the denial.

When the severity of the illness can no longer be denied, a natural reaction to realizing that one's life is about to end is intense anger, even rage, along with envy and resentment. It is very clear where the anger comes from. Life is being shortened prematurely from cancer, everything the patient has known and loved must end, and the future that was anticipated will never happen. A terminally ill patient might behave in uncharacteristic ways, becoming cantankerous, critical, abusive, and aggressive, finding grievances everywhere and lashing out at anyone trying to help. His anger might be displaced in any direction, projected out into the environment almost at random. He might be angry at medical personnel, family members, or anyone around him who is healthy and can expect to enjoy life in ways that he himself no longer will. Whether the anger is rational or not, family members would do well to try not to take it personally. Even when it is aimed at them, usually they are not the real target. There might be no one else with whom the patient feels safe enough to express his anger, frustration, helplessness, or any kind of distress.

Sometimes, when there is no strength left for anger, depression sets in. At times there is a sense of agonizing loss, loneliness, anguish, and despair that destroys all joy. Time is running out and there is no way out. Losses in the past—mistakes made, goals never achieved, decisions and actions regretted—can never be changed. The future holds the loss of everything and everyone the dying person has known and loved, as well as her dreams of what might be. While family members can discuss with the patient the past losses, pointing out the brighter side of things that have happened, the prospect of losing everything is wordless. There are no words, but the presence of loved ones and their touch can bring some comfort. Here it is particularly true that pain shared is pain lessened.

People who are dying often also feel fear. They might be afraid of being in intolerable pain, of suffering, of dying, and of death itself. They might be frightened when they think about the effects their death will have on the people they love. When the person is afraid, the family can try to be there with him as he needs them.

Acceptance is not always a serene or necessarily transformative state, neither is it one that is always reached. It is simply the recognition that nothing can be done to change what is happening. It is the time when the patient realizes that treating the illness is pointless and that she is powerless against death, and so stops struggling.

Meeting the Patient's Needs

The family can demonstrate and express their love by trying to meet the patient's greatest needs and thus ease her process of dying. Her most immediate need is to have distressing physical problems addressed. She also needs to feel valued and not alone, connected to people with whom she can talk honestly, who can listen to her fears and concerns and understand them. She needs to control her life in whatever ways she can. She needs to come to some understanding of the meaning of her life, and, finally, she needs a sense of completion.

Family members can offer all these things. Many focus only on the patient's physical needs and ignore the others. After physical needs are met, what the patient needs most is that her family members be there with her, available to her emotionally.

The Need to Communicate—or Not

Being there involves attentive listening. Asking the patient what she is thinking or feeling can sometimes help, but she might not want to answer. Some people who are dying turn inward, sometimes out of the need to begin separating from everyone and everything. Being present with her involves allowing her to talk about whatever she wishes to or not to talk at all. The point is to let her be where she is, not where anyone thinks she should be. The best thing to do is to let her express her wishes about what to talk about and whom to talk with. Just to sit with her and allow her to be quiet is a great gift. People need to die in their own way, just as they need to live in their own way.

Some patients want to talk about death and dying, some don't. Some caregivers, apparently influenced by popular literature, have the idea that the person who is dying ought to be talking about it. They worry if the patient hasn't brought up the subject (even when the patient is just very sick and not near death at all). This is completely misguided. The only things the person ought to be talking about are whatever she wants to, and for some people that does not include discussions about death. Some patients do want to talk about it, but not necessarily with the people closest to them. It can be helpful for the patient to be asked if she would like to talk with a clergyperson or pastoral counselor. If she does, the family must understand that any such conversations are private unless the patient chooses to tell them what was said.

Often someone who is seriously ill wants to explore what it means to be dying, and to express her wishes about a future of which she will no longer be a part. Some family members do not allow the patient to share their innermost thoughts and feelings, perhaps because they can't bear to hear them. Their unwillingness deprives everyone.

A family member might well ask her therapist, "What do I say if he [the patient] asks if he's dying?" One answer to this client might be, "You might say, 'I can tell you what the doctors said. But first tell me, what would it mean to you if you were dying, and what would it mean if you weren't?'"

When the patient and family can share their concerns, their regrets, their unresolved feelings, and their sense of loss, fear, and loneliness at the impending separation, this can bring them closer together, comfort them, and strengthen them. When their communication is fruitful, their self-knowledge can grow and their relationships deepen. Once they can talk openly about what they are feeling and thinking, they can spend their time together far more creatively, productively, and lovingly.

Their communication might well take many forms. Whatever form it takes, it does not cease to be important and fruitful, even when the end is nearing. At that time, family members might sit near the patient, often for hours at a time, while the patient dozes or lies quietly. To communicate that they care, it is not necessary that they do anything other than to be there or nearby. There is no need for them to say anything except in response to the patient. For the patient, to open her eyes to see a loved one sitting there says and means everything. The family member might ask from time to time if there is anything the patient might like to discuss. If there is, the family member would do well to listen. Even if the patient repeats the same things again and again, or if what she says is unintelligible or doesn't make sense, whatever she says is communication. Family members can communicate with their touch, offering to hold her hand, stroke her arm, or massage her hands or feet. Words are not needed. Their touch can bring comfort, connection, and security. Even in the last moments of our lives, none of us wants to be alone.

The Need for Autonomy: Choices About Living

People are either alive or dead. As long as we are alive, we need to do what we are capable of doing and to participate in decisions about how we live during the remaining months, weeks, or days of our lives. This is what dying with dignity means: maintaining autonomy, the ability to make choices during one's last days.

Family members often tend to try to protect the patient by taking away his autonomy. This is antithetical to being supportive. It is a great mistake for anyone to deprive someone who is ill of doing anything that the person can do for himself. The family can help enormously by encouraging the patient to identify what he can still do and wants to do, and to respond to those choices. There might be things he wants to accomplish, activities he wants to undertake, projects he wants to work on, people he wants to see or communicate with, things he wants to talk about, or places he wants to see. He might want to consider what complementary therapies he wants to pursue, or what kind of support he wants as his situation worsens. Perhaps he wants to prepare for his death or to spend time with friends or family. Many people obtain comfort from returning to their religious roots at the end of their lives. In whatever ways possible, the family can help to maximize the patient's quality of life in whatever ways are meaningful to him, and to provide him with a sense of control, purpose, and accomplishment during whatever time remains.

As the patient grows weaker and more dependent, his sphere of choice slowly diminishes. One of his greatest emotional needs at this time is to retain control in whatever areas of life it is still possible to do so. If he is at home, this means having control over such matters as when to eat, what to eat, whom to talk with, how long visits should be, having a pet on the bed, or seeing and touching children in the family.

The patient might find himself sent to a nursing home or care facility without having a say about where he is going, or in a hospital where tests and procedures are being done that he neither understands nor wants. Such experiences are hardly conducive to his making decisions about his life and destiny. Even in those situations, however, some choices remain, and family members can help greatly by maximizing them. They can try to respond to the patient's wishes and to avoid anything that does not accord with his wishes or that causes discomfort. They can respect his need for control in every area possible. Even small choices can make a difference to his feeling of self-worth. ("Joe is on the phone. Do you want to talk to him or shall I ask him to call back later?" "Here's the juice you asked for. Would you like some now?" "Is this the blanket you wanted?")

The Need for Autonomy: Choices About Dying

Cancer usually gives everyone in the family time to prepare for death. When the patient has accepted the fact that her life is about to end, then she can make plans and decisions for that eventuality that make it possible for her remaining time to be as satisfying and comforting as it can be. The patient has the opportunity to make decisions that carry the weight of her own authority, not medical authority. Preparing for the patient's death can be important for the entire family's peace of mind.

Drawing up a will, communicating what she wants done with her assets and possessions, can bring reassurance that her loved ones will be cared for when she is gone and ease the prospect of dying. The patient might also be reassured by discussing with her family members how they will manage and how the family will go on. Some people have clear ideas about what they want in regard to their funeral, memorial services, and burial or cremation. They should be given the opportunity to express their wishes about these matters.

Many people find peace of mind by arranging for legal directives concerning their medical care for the time when death approaches. A living will provides assurance to patients that only those medical interventions that they have specified will be performed. A durable power of attorney for health care (health care proxy) names someone to make decisions about treatment and care should the patient be unable to do so. A power of attorney names someone to sign medical, financial, or legal documents if the patient is unable to do so. All these documents assure the dying person that her wishes will be carried out. (Appendix 6 describes these documents in more detail.)

All such arrangements for putting affairs in order help to meet patients' need to finish unfinished business and complete their lives.

The Need for Meaning and Completion

All of us need to understand the meaning of our lives before we die. We need to know what it was all about so that we can have a sense of completeness within ourselves and in relationship to others. We need to look back on our experiences, bring them together, and see them as an integrated whole, to determine whether they had value and meaning. We want to know that our life made a difference to someone, and that we accomplished something. We want to have our life affirmed (Hudson, 1990). We cannot really say goodbye to anything without knowing what it was. Before we take leave of life, we need to know ourselves.

The patient's feelings of isolation and loneliness can be eased considerably by family members or others who can help him find meaning in his life and thus complete it in his own way and on his own terms. Some patients might be helped in this by being encouraged to complete a project they had begun, or to talk with people with whom they feel there is too much still left unsaid. Some people create meaning before they die by leaving some kind of a legacy reflecting their values, such as a letter to their children or some kind of a contribution to others. Sometimes simply focusing on the good things they enjoy and appreciate, or even just getting out of bed for a while, can bring meaning to their life.

Although family members are not trained therapists, hospice workers, or pastoral counselors, they can help the patient look at his life as a whole by discussing what was most meaningful to him. The patient might begin by remembering and revisiting his roots and considering what shaped him. The family can look at photographs together and share life stories and family history. They can initiate dialogues in which they ask the patient such questions as, "What has your life been like for you?" "What were some of the best moments?" "What were some of the hardest?" "What moments in your life are you the most proud of?" "What do you most regret?" "What would you change if you could?" "For those decisions you regret, what do you need to do now to be able to forgive yourself?" (For more of such questions, see *Cancer as a Turning Point*, LeShan, 1994, chapter 8). Very often, once these conversations can begin, they start to flow. When this kind of dialogue is fruitful, even at this time the patient can grow in self-knowledge.

The family can meet the patient's need for meaning in another way as well: They can give him the assurance that he has been loved. They can tell him about the ways he has had an impact on their lives, remind him of times he helped them, and express what he has meant to them. When they can do this, the patient knows that he will continue to live in their memories, and they themselves will have few regrets about what they have left unsaid.

In all these ways, family members deepen their relationships with the patient and complete for themselves their time with him. Hopefully, in the future they can tell themselves, "I have done all that I could."

CHAPTER 14

How Family Caregivers Can Best Help Themselves

If I am not for myself, who will be for me?
If I am only for myself, what am I?
And if not now, when?
Rabbi Hillel, *The Talmud, Ethics of the Fathers*

Many family caregivers need to be reminded again and again that it is their right as well as their responsibility to take care of themselves. They often ignore their own needs, drop everything they enjoy and care about, and focus only on the person who is ill. Insofar as they forget that caring and giving to others need to be balanced with caring and giving to themselves, they are certain to burn out.

The idea of taking time for themselves might make them feel guilty, particularly if the patient is not getting better and needs more care. Yet unless they give themselves permission to take the time to maintain their strength and to relax for a while, they do their entire family a disservice.

Fuel makes a car go, but the car cannot go anywhere unless the fuel is continually replenished. Similarly, if family caregivers fail to take care of their own physical and mental health, they are certain to become so physically and emotionally drained that they will be unable to help anyone else when they are most needed.

It is essential that family caregivers be sensitive to their own health and well-being while being sensitive to the patients' needs. They need to understand that only by giving themselves permission to take care of themselves will they be able to provide continued help and support to the person who is ill over the course of the illness and treatment.

For Caregivers: Ways to Help Yourself

1. You have a responsibility to take care of your physical health and well-being.

All too often, many people caring for family members who are ill don't eat enough, or don't eat balanced meals, or overeat. Too often they don't get enough sleep, exercise, or relaxation. Very often they neglect their health and are overdue for routine physical care. For these reasons they are at particular risk for physical problems.

Therefore, it is important that you eat regularly, planning for your own nutritional needs as carefully as you do for those of the patient. It is just as important that you try to get enough sleep. Physical exercise, even just daily walks, can help you feel better emotionally and physically. It is highly advisable that you see a physician for a complete physical exam and that you keep up with medical checkups.

2. Taking care of your emotional health and well-being involves making time just for yourself.

You need to be involved in activities other than caregiving. You need rest, relaxation, recreation, and pleasure. You have a right to tell the patient and others that you are tired and need to rest, or that you need a break from the routine to pursue activities you enjoy outside the home. You have a right to say that you need to take care of yourself so that you can care for others.

Try to take time at least once a week to maintain your interests and do things you enjoy and care about, with others or alone. Your activities might include pursuing a hobby, joining a health club, taking a class, or going somewhere to relax with friends who make you feel good about yourself and with whom you can laugh and talk. They might include going to a concert, seeing a movie, or just sitting quietly and watching the grass grow.

3. With the patient, make plans for the future.

Cancer can make people forget that there is a future. Develop short-term goals and long-term visions. Approach this planning optimistically and realistically, keeping in mind the patient's limitations and everyone's interests. For example, you might want to start planning long or short trips by discussing where you would most like to go, reading travel guides and brochures, and even buying tickets. Your plans need to be flexible. (You can buy travel insurance along with tickets.) You might want to learn to make wine in your basement, study Etruscan art, or see a circus. Whatever plans you make, carry them out as often as possible. To paraphrase Goethe, whatever you can do, or dream you can, begin it now.

4. Accept or enlist all the help you can get.

Caregivers often take on more than they can handle, and in some situations this is not always necessary. You might well discover that you can be more effective and productive if you delegate some tasks. Older children can help with housecleaning or cooking. (It helps them to help.) Friends, relatives, and neighbors who offer to help can be given tasks that fit their abilities and schedules, even it is simply accompanying the patient to a medical appointment. If you are not comfortable leaving the patient home alone, ask one of them to stay for a while so you can get out for a few hours.

When necessary, consider hiring someone to help. Options include hiring a temporary home health aide. It might be possible to hire a neighborhood college or high school student inexpensively to help with tasks you dislike or don't have time for, or just to buy some time to relax.

Seek out sources of support from cancer organizations and local cancer support groups. You can also find information on the Internet, at the Family Caregiver Alliance Web site: www.caregiver.org.

5. *You have a right to defend and protect yourself.*

Although it is very natural for anyone with cancer to feel frustration and anger, even rage, this does not mean that you have to tolerate abuse or violence. The patient might accuse you of not doing enough or not doing things right. If the patient lashes out at you, try to ignore the accusations and defuse the situation. ("The way you're talking to me is not okay. Let's talk about this later, when we can do it calmly. Right now I'm too upset." "It scares me when you talk that way. I love you and don't want to fight with you. Can we discuss this quietly?") There is no reason to allow yourself to be abused, and you need to say so.

6. *You need to learn how to handle other people's insensitivity or unsolicited advice.*

Some stock responses you may find useful include: "Thanks for the idea. I'll consider it." "I appreciate your thinking of us, but I need to do this my way." "I don't know if that is what [the patient] wants. I'll ask him."

7. *Find outside sources of emotional support.*

Besides your friends and your therapist, you might find it helpful to explore cancer organizations and their support groups. Classes in yoga, exercise, or relaxation techniques might also be helpful. (Appendix 4 describes some techniques for managing stress.)

An Exercise for Caregivers

Try writing your responses to all the parts of this exercise (LeShan, 1994).

1. Suppose someone who loved you unconditionally gave you a special gift: a block of time. There is one catch, one string attached: You must use the time only for yourself, for your own growth or enjoyment or well-being. What would you do?

2. Realistically, is there a block of time you can arrange to take for yourself, once every week or even two weeks? The time might be scheduled regularly (for example, every Wednesday afternoon) or irregularly (3 or 4 hours at one time or other during the week). Can you be as kind to yourself as you would be to someone else who loves you?

3. Will you arrange this time for yourself: yes or no? If your answer was no, what stops you? Usually what stops us is something inside ourselves, not external situations. If your answer was yes, why haven't you taken this time for yourself sooner?

CHAPTER 15

Afterward

. . . No life lives for ever;
. . . Even the weariest river
Winds somewhere safe to sea.
Algernon Swinburne, "The Garden of Proserpine"

Most people battling cancer win. More patients than ever before are pronounced cancer free after treatment. Both these patients and their family members may well have many emotional reactions when treatment ends—and for a long time afterward. Often it is only after their fight has ended that they can afford to take in fully how difficult and frightening it has been. They are also likely to begin harboring new fears about the possibility of a rediagnosis in the future. Continuing checkups, even years later, can bring back memories of the dark times and incite fears of another diagnosis. Slowly with time these fears ease, and with more time, they usually recede.

Some cancer patients do not survive. Their family members, who have been watching time get away from them, suddenly find that time is gone. "We say that the hour of death cannot be forecast," Marcel Proust wrote in *Remembrance of Things Past*, "but we imagine that hour as placed in an obscure and distant future. It never occurs to us that it has any connection with the day already begun."

Even when the patient was not expected to live, those who love him are never prepared to lose him. After the death, surviving family members who were intimately involved with the patient's illness and dying might feel that a part of them has died, too. They are likely to go through all the emotions they experienced earlier—but now with an intensity perhaps never before experienced, and now without hope. C. S. Lewis, writing of his grief after his beloved wife died of cancer, said that the pain he felt now was part of his happiness then, and "that's the deal."

The Many Faces of Grief

No matter how long someone has been a caregiver, the finality of the patient's death is likely to be grasped slowly. Denial now is again protective, offering respite from time to time from the pain of loss. Family members might need to recount the story of the death over and over again until they can take in its truth.

Their anger might seem boundless, directed at the patient for leaving them, at themselves for not preventing the death, at doctors, God, the universe, anyone close to them, or anyone else. Like denial, their anger is protective, offering for a little while purpose and energy that is far more tolerable than the nothingness of deep loss. They might feel regret at decisions made or not made during the last days that they think might have made the patient's life better or easier in some ways.

At the same time they might feel relief—along with guilt for feeling it. They have poured time and energy, heart and soul, love and compassion into the battle with cancer. For as long as the patient was ill, cancer took over their lives. Their own pain was made heavier watching the patient's suffering. Now the patient's pain has ended, his suffering has ended, and death has ended the disease. In view of all this, it is hardly surprising or terrible that reactions to the patient's death might be "Thank God it's over at last!" and "I'm free." Feelings of relief are as natural to family caregivers as they are to a soldier returning home after a war. They might have been living for weeks or months with the dispiriting knowledge that there was only one way the battle could end (Pomeroy, 1996). They might also feel guilt because they are alive and the patient is not.

Before the death occurs, caregivers have already done a lot of grieving. During all the time the patient was not getting better, as they watched him no longer able to do things that he had always done, as they saw his emotional and physical pain, most family members felt anticipatory grief. They grieved long before the patient's life was lost, as they watched it slowing, headed nowhere. Whatever grief they have already felt will not necessarily make their mourning shorter or longer now (Kübler-Ross & Kessler, 2005).

The patient's death brings many losses. Family members have lost the person they knew and loved, and the life they had. They have lost the part of themselves that was in relationship to the patient: They are no longer a husband or wife, sibling, adult child, or parent. They have lost the future they expected. Often their loss destroys the foundation on which they base their understanding of the world, which might include their faith in a God who brings meaning or their belief that life has meaning at all.

Every death we experience is tied to every other. The patient's death might well evoke grief for losses in the past that were not fully mourned.

Along with grief, family members might well feel vulnerability, isolation, and depression that they believe will never end. Many of them believe that they cannot live without the person who has died, and that their lives will never be whole and fulfilling again. Their days seem empty, aimless, and disorganized.

Therapists are cautioned again to be aware that this depression, no matter how deep, is normal. Unlike clinical depressive conditions, the depression following loss involves specific sorrows that the client can readily identify. The use of antidepressant medications for those clients is a controversial issue, one that needs to be considered carefully for each individual by a medical professional who knows the client and the situation (Kübler-Ross & Kessler, 2005).

Depression and grief disrupt normal physical functions. All the changes in lifestyle caused by the patient's absence disrupt the hormonal, immune, nervous, and cardiovascular systems. These changes can lead to such symptoms as impaired concentration, weakness, fatigue, sleeplessness, loss of appetite, and resultant weight loss (Holland & Lewis, 2001).

Acceptance is coming to terms with the reality that the patient's death is final and that surviving family members must learn to live with it. It takes as long it takes to get to that place. There are no timetables.

How the Therapist Can Help

All deaths are not the same. All mourning is not the same. Some losses leave wounds that never fully heal. There are no right ways to mourn, no systematic progressions through stages of grief, and no schedules or deadlines for the pain of loss to ease. Life will never return to what was normal for the family member, for it will never again be the same.

Clients who come to their therapists in grief need to talk about the dying and the death, sometimes again and again. Talking about what happened helps them to believe that it has happened. They need to express their grief and pain, and be heard. They might also need to express regret—about things done or not done, said or not said, or for all that will remain incomplete. The therapist can encourage this simply with questions.

Whatever emotion the client feels, it is vital that it be accepted. It is a serious mistake to try to divert someone's pain by telling him he should not feel what he feels and urging him to be in a different emotional place than where he is. It is never helpful to urge clients who mourn not to be angry or sad, or not to have regrets. It is just as great a mistake to offer false reassurance or to predict how they are going to feel. They must be allowed to experience, without limitations, whatever tangle of feelings and thoughts assaults them at this time. They are helped most by those who can simply sit with them and listen. The therapist's main task at this time is just to be there, be supportive, and encourage the client to talk. That is the most we can do.

After their initial shock and mourning, clients will need months or years to adapt to living without the person they loved and begin rebuilding their lives. There is no schedule, no date by which they can be expected to get on with their lives. Losing a loved one, often along with a faith in God or in a universe that is fair and meaningful, can send anyone adrift in despair. These losses do not disappear but with time usually they ease.

It can be helpful for therapists to tell their clients that they will never fully get over their loss, but that although their pain will still hurt, it will come less often. It is also helpful to point out that they are in deep grief because of their deep love and later, as their grief lessens, this does not mean that they loved any less.

Every person responds to grief and eases his pain in his own way. Some find healing through some kind of memorial to remember and honor the person they lost, such as memorial rituals or contributions to organizations in the person's name. Some find solace in being with others who have shared the loss. Some deal with their loss simply by their involvement in day-to-day life in the present. Many create meaning by using their experiences to volunteer to help others. Whatever ways they plan for themselves are to be encouraged. (The exception is that these clients should be cautioned not to do any volunteer work with cancer patients for at least a year or until they know they are strong enough to handle it.)

Therapists can encourage clients to take advantage of sources of support available to them: friends, relatives, clergy, and the therapists themselves. Family members might need to be reminded that those who were close to the patient can provide comfort and strength to one another as they share their grief. The client might also want to investigate support groups, whose members all understand full well what the others are experiencing.

Each of us is changed forever by the experience of loss and grief of someone we loved, to whom we were deeply connected. The depth of our pain reflects the depth of our love. Difficult as it is to endure, grief sometimes serves some useful purposes. It slows us down and allows us to assess our loss. It can force us to rebuild ourselves and our lives. It can bring us to a deeper place that we might not normally explore (Kübler-Ross & Kessler, 2005). It leads us to a kind of growth, maturity, and strength that we did not know before. We never forget the person we loved to whom we were closely connected. Although we are never again the same, we survive and somehow find our way back to involvement with life and living. Everyone needs to find their own ways through their mourning—and most people do.

Epilogue: Preventing Burnout and Discovering Unexpected Gifts

"Understanding" means "standing under the same sky and sharing the same world."

Jacob Needleman (personal communication
to Lawrence LeShan, April 16, 1964)

The problem with clients dealing with cancer is that they make us anxious. When they invite us to share their deep emotional pain, sometimes we fear that if we accept this invitation, we could absorb their suffering.

Some therapists apparently believe that working with such clients is something like performing cardiopulmonary resuscitation. When you learn to perform CPR, you are instructed to keep going until one of three things happens: (a) the victim, who has been unconscious, moves, in which case he doesn't need your help any longer; (b) another rescuer arrives to relieve you; or (c) you are too exhausted to continue.

Is this anything like your idea of how it is to work with family caregivers? Are you afraid that you will keep taking in their pain until you are too exhausted to continue? After someone close to them is diagnosed with cancer, some clients begin to believe that life is simply a series of sufferings. Are you concerned that by being exposed to their seemingly unrelieved distress, you would lose your perspective and come to believe that, too?

In one of the most significant times of their lives, people dealing with cancer come to us in pain. When they talk about their lives, we become all too aware that someone dear to us or even we ourselves could be diagnosed, too. When they express their helplessness at not being able to fix the person they love, we might feel helpless because we don't know how to fix them. They might feel guilty because they are well while someone close to them is suffering in ways that they are not. We might feel guilty because they are suffering in ways that we are not. When they express their emotional distress, they touch our own wounds, old losses, and fears. When they talk about death and dying, they remind us that that will happen to us, too. Their darkness is no different from what might be waiting for us. They threaten us because they are our mirrors.

So it is tempting and natural to defend ourselves by building emotional barriers, walls of professional detachment and programmed techniques and responses, to keep their pain from touching us so we won't get hurt or burn out. Nothing in our professional code of ethics specifically prohibits this. Our training might even have encouraged us to insulate ourselves from direct encounters with our clients, and we might believe that it is for their benefit or the benefit of our work together that we do so. Besides, even when we are aware that we put up walls, we tell ourselves that our clients don't know the walls are there.

There are several major problems with this. One is that these clients turn to us because they want to be with caring human beings, not technicians. We can't help them unless we stay present with them. When we erect walls to keep them at a distance, we lose our most valuable therapeutic assets: our own emotions and our personal experiences. Unless we are open to our own losses, suffering, and pain, we can't be open to theirs, and we can't help them. Our willingness to allow ourselves to be openly human is precisely what connects us to them. It is also what makes it possible for them to trust us.

The walls we put up are not invisible. We are mistaken when we think that clients don't know they are there. When we try to keep out their pain and our own, we also keep these clients out. With our practiced behavior and automatic comments, we fail them. We cannot meet their need to look deep inside themselves to find understanding and meaning in what is happening in their lives. "If the therapist has reservations about meeting the patient fully, the patient senses it and it reinforces his reservations about meeting life and meeting himself" (Bowers et al., 1964, p. 86).

The greatest problem with trying to protect ourselves by distancing is that it almost guarantees that we will burn out. The emotions that these clients can evoke in us that we don't want to feel don't disappear. Like any suppressed feelings, they just fester, grow, and distort.

Besides, erecting and maintaining walls requires effort and energy that we can use far more productively in other ways—particularly when these barriers aren't really necessary at all. We can be with our clients and respond in a genuine way without losing ourselves. It is not always easy to strike a balance between being professionally and personally involved—but it is possible. It is surely a goal worth striving for. So how can we manage to do this?

First, we can try to be our authentic selves. When we aren't, we'll soon know it. If we hear ourselves mouthing phrases or using techniques that we've practiced, if our voice sounds odd to ourselves, or if our clients seem to be listening politely rather than being engaged, those are clues we can respond to. If we find ourselves unusually fatigued after a session, this is also a clue. Being authentic means setting aside our fears and letting ourselves be genuine, rather than distancing behind a professional façade. It means seeing the client as a human being much like ourselves, so that we can react with understanding and compassion. At times, for example, authenticity involves laughing when that comes naturally. (People dealing with cancer usually don't have enough opportunities to laugh and welcome it when it can happen.) It might also involve crying with them when that comes naturally.

Another thing we can do is to remind ourselves (as often as necessary) that we can't change our clients' situations. We want to make them feel better. We want to fix them, but our task is to help them be where they are, not where we think they should be. We cannot take away their suffering. We cannot rescue them, and they did not come to us to be rescued. Our task is to be there—really be there. We aren't required to say much. (Most therapists learn, usually the hard way, that if we don't know what to say, it's far better to say nothing.) For these clients who are dealing every day with a life crisis, talking relieves much anxiety and being heard is a gift we give them. As one therapist said, we don't need to have the answers, just to share the questions (Lochner, 1990a).

We also need to nourish ourselves in all the ways we advise our clients to do. Beginning with our physical health, we need to consciously examine all the facets of our own being from time to time—physical, mental, emotional, relational, creative, and spiritual—to determine whether any has been neglected and needs care. To use LeShan's phrase, we need to develop and actively maintain "a fierce and tender concern for all of ourselves" (1994, p. 158). What do we want from our life? How can we live so that our life reflects who we are? What do we need to change or add so that each day becomes more meaningful, exciting, and fulfilling? We need to honor every aspect of our own being. We cannot be there for our clients when we are too physically or emotionally tired because we haven't cared for ourselves and our own lives. By neglecting ourselves, in effect we say to our clients, "Do as I say, not as I do."

Clearly, to work with these people, there is much personal processing we have to tend to inside ourselves. We all have had losses in our life. We can be with these clients as they need us to be only if we have faced our own fears, pain, anger, grief, and despair, and accept our own feelings. We need to look at the mystery of death and confront the reality of our own mortality. Charles Lochner, who teaches professional courses on death and dying, wrote that after we read all the professional books and finish all the training and workshops, we still have to confront death, both our own and others'. The task is to look within ourselves at our own lives, our own suffering, and our own daily dying. Without doing this, we cannot be fully present with anyone. Without owning our own pain we will be frightened by the pain of others (Lochner, 1990b).

Being open to our own losses, our own suffering, and our own mortality is not the easiest thing for anyone to do, but unless we do that, we cannot be open to clients who live with that reality every day. Unless we do that, we will bring our own issues into our work with them—and then we will surely burn out.

Clearly, to look within ourselves and to face all that we meet in our clients, we need to do an enormous amount of homework. Homework includes many years of personal therapy as well as supervision. No matter how much therapy we have already had, no matter how old or how experienced we are, when we work with people dealing with life-threatening illness, we need our own therapist. As long as we work with clients who can so easily push all our buttons, we also need a supervisor. The therapist and supervisor may or may not be the same person, for there is a fine line between supervision dealing with our work with these clients and therapy dealing with what they evoke in us.

In view of all the difficulties, why would any therapist want to work with people dealing with cancer? Why would we want to engage with people trying to cope with crisis or tragedy every day? Why would you? As another way to prevent burnout, it is helpful for therapists to ask ourselves that question and explore the answers. It is one of the most important questions we can ask ourselves. You are likely to find that you have a number of different answers. Some probably relate to your own life experiences and the effects they have had on you. Some might have to do with the meaning you make of them. Some might have to do with your sense of who you are. One of your reasons for wanting to do this work might be simply that you know that you can. (If you don't know this, if you doubt that you can deal with these clients' pain, then it might be a good idea to refer them to someone else.)

Profound and Unexpected Gifts

Without doubt this work is extremely challenging, but at the same time it brings unexpected rewards that make it deeply fulfilling.

In our training as therapists, we were taught that we show our clients the way by personal modeling. That is, by demonstrating our willingness to enter into a deep and honest emotional relationship with them, we can change their feelings about themselves and they can then change the way they are with others. What is not usually mentioned is that people who come to therapy because of cancer in their lives often serve as models for us. Being with them often teaches us some important things.

We learn by trying that we can be ourselves and stay open with our clients, no matter what they express, without losing who we are. From this we find that we can stay open with people who are not our clients.

People dealing with cancer have their own priorities straight. They usually know what is important to them, and most are honest and direct. When we put aside our fears to allow ourselves to feel whatever we feel with them, we usually find that we are not drained or depleted, as we might have imagined. We are enlivened. Their honesty, their openness, and their depth of feeling often move us and energize us. As a result, we are better able to vitalize them.

We learn a lot about living. Being with these clients sharpens our sensitivity to life and its preciousness.

We learn from them a great deal about what it means to be a human being. In them we see a profound sense of life and deep feelings. Their despair, sorrow, and fear often go hand in hand with honesty, determination, strength, courage, and dignity. We see their deep altruism and commitment, and their capacity for humor and love that can light even the darkest times (Bowers et al., 1964). We come to respect them greatly, for they show us what human beings can be.

They give us the opportunity to contribute to life.

The physician Eric Cassell (1994) wrote that seasoned practitioners who care for people dealing with critical illness learn from direct experience that the more completely open and unconcerned with self-protection they are, the less the emotional price of caring and the greater the rewards. He added, however, that it takes time to learn this.

When I first began my training and years of supervision with Larry LeShan, knowing that all his early clinical research had been conducted with patients who were terminally ill, I asked him, "How do you deal with all this?" His answer was brief and simple. "You cry a lot," he said. I came to learn that in fact this is the only way. As I tell my clients, you can't turn off feelings selectively. You can't choose to feel some emotions and not others. Either you feel or you don't. Our capacity for pain and hurt is our capacity for joy and compassion.

Anyone doing this work needs to be very involved with living. A new oncology nurse, Theresa Brown, wrote about her experience when, for the first time, a patient she was caring for died. Her words would be well heeded by therapists and any health professionals trying to help people dealing with a life-threatening illness:

> What can one do? Go home, love your children, try not to bicker, eat well, walk in the rain, feel the sun on your face and laugh loud and often, as much as possible, and especially at yourself. Because the only antidote to death is not poetry or drama or miracles or a roomful of technical expertise and good intentions. The antidote to death is life. (Brown, 2008, p. F1)

To be present with clients in crisis and help them requires us to have a passion for life and living. This involves accepting life on its own terms, in its totality, with all its contradictions, complete with illness, pain and loneliness, joy and laughter, death and dying. When we can do this, we find that life is indeed the antidote.

Some Basic Facts About Cancer

What Cancer Is

The word *cancer* refers to more than 100 diseases that can occur in any part of the body. What they all have in common is the uncontrolled growth and multiplication of abnormal cells that can spread (metastasize).

The human body is made of billions of cells, its building blocks, which form tissues. Cells take in nutrients, grow, and divide to reproduce as the body requires. Each new cell is the exact genetic copy of the one from which it came. When cells grow old, new cells are created to replace them. Every second, millions of cells are created while millions of others die. Normally cell reproduction and growth follows an orderly pattern: cells are born, they live for a certain amount of time, and they die. The body has a control mechanism to maintain a balance, so that the numbers of cells that die are roughly equal to those replacing them.

Sometimes, however, the control mechanism fails to function normally, so that the balance is no longer maintained. There is an uncontrolled growth of new cells that the body does not need. Cells divide in unpredictable, rampant ways, and old cells do not die when they should. The extra cells form a mass of tissues, a growth (tumor).

As the cells keep multiplying out of control, they form larger and larger tumors. Unlike normal cells that are cohesive, these uncontrolled cells are loose and can detach from one another. When they detach, they do not always die. They do what normal cells cannot do: they move around and spread. Because they are minuscule, they can be carried in the bloodstream or the lymph system to close or distant parts of the body, invading local tissues, nearby structures, or distant organs, forming new tumors there. As they reproduce, they can displace normal tissues, causing obstructions. They can invade any part of the body. No tissue, not even bone, is immune. It is the spread that is life threatening. If it is not stopped, and these cells invade vital organs, they can overwhelm the body, crowding out normal tissue and causing symptoms leading to death. Such tumors, made up of uncontrolled cells, are cancerous (malignant).

Some tumors, although they are abnormal growths, do not reproduce uncontrollably, nor do they spread to tissues around them or to other parts of the body. These are not cancerous; they are benign.

The original mass is called the primary tumor. Every cancer is defined and named for its primary site. When cells spread to a different location, they have the same composition and the same name as the primary tumor. For example, if breast cancer spreads to the bones, those cancer cells in the bones are breast cancer cells. The condition would be regarded as metastatic breast cancer rather than bone cancer.

Causes

There are numerous theories about the cause of cancer, having to do with something going wrong with the immune system so that it no longer destroys aberrant cells. However, the exact cause of any individual's cancer is not known. The disease appears to be due to some combination of genetic, environmental, and, to some unknown extent, psychological factors.

Classifications

Tumors are characterized and classified in different ways. The classification determines the medical treatment and also suggests the prognosis.

Site: Types of Cell and Organs

Most malignant tumors fall into six main groups, depending on their site of origin and their structure. No one type is more prevalent or more dangerous than any other, and any of them can spread locally or to more distant parts of the body.

Carcinoma, the most common kind, occurs in cells that form glands covering the body's surface or lining internal organs. Cancers of the breast, colon, rectum, female reproductive system, lung, prostate, and skin are all carcinomas.

Sarcoma originates in the connective or supportive tissues anywhere in the body: in muscles, bones, cartilage, tendons, nerves, and blood vessels.

Leukemia develops in the tissues that form blood cells: the bone marrow, lymph nodes, and spleen.

Lymphoma originates in the cells of the lymph symptom. Hodgkin's disease is one kind of lymphoma; all other types are referred to as non-Hodgkin's lymphomas.

Blastoma originates in embryonic tissue of organs.

Myeloma originates in bone marrow.

Differentiation

Cancer is also classified by how quickly a tumor is likely to grow, which is determined by examining specimens taken from the tumor. Cells of a well-differentiated tumor appear under a microscope much like those of the normal tissue from where they were taken. Cells of an undifferentiated tumor appear different from those of the normal tissue that surrounded it. Undifferentiated tumors are more aggressive—that is, they grow faster and spread sooner.

Grades

Another classification system, mainly for sarcomas and brain tumors, has to do with the extent of abnormality. It grades tumors on a scale of 1 to 4: The greater the extent of abnormality, the higher the grade. A high-grade tumor is immature, undifferentiated, and fast growing. A low-grade tumor is differentiated and slower growing.

Stages

Based on information about type and behavior of the tumor, pathologists evaluate and classify the severity on a scale of 0 to 4, according to how large it is and how far the cancer has spread. It is usually the stage of the tumor that determines the treatment.

- Stage I tumors are small and have not spread.
- Stage II tumors are larger than those in Stage I, and might have spread to nearby lymph nodes.
- Stage III tumors have grown more than Stage II tumors, and usually have spread to nearby lymph nodes.
- Stage IV tumors have grown and spread even more widely, usually having invaded other organs.

Sources

Alpha Institute. (1993). *The Alpha book on cancer and living.* Alameda, CA: Author.

American Cancer Society and CURE. (2008). *Cancer resource guide.* Dallas, TX: Susan McClure.

Balch, C. (Ed.). (2008). *Cancer guide: A treatment and facilities guide for patients and their families.* Parkville, MO: Patient Resource Publishing.

Coleman, C. N. (2006). *Understanding cancer.* Baltimore, MD: Johns Hopkins University Press.

Geffen, G. (2006). *The journey through cancer.* New York: Three Rivers Press.

Laszlo, J. (1988). *Understanding cancer.* New York: Harper and Row.

Some Basic Facts About Cancer Treatments

Different types of cancer might behave very differently, growing at different rates and responding to different treatments. For that reason, patients need treatments aimed at their particular kind of cancer.

Every family in which someone has been diagnosed with cancer is faced with a confusing array of treatment choices, ranging from sophisticated, cutting-edge medical treatments to outright dangerous or at least ineffectual popular philosophies.

There are three main categories of treatments:

1. Conventional (mainstream, standard, or orthodox) medical treatments, whose effectiveness has been studied and demonstrated by medical science;
2. Complementary (adjunctive or adjuvant) treatments, used in conjunction with medical treatment; and
3. Alternative treatments, used in place of conventional treatment.

Conventional Medical Treatments

Medical treatment can have any of three goals:

1. To cure the illness. For cancer, a cure means that no signs or symptoms remain (the disease is in remission) for a specified number of years after treatment, indicating that all the cancer cells have been destroyed. The specific period of remission varies depending on the kind of cancer.
2. To manage or control the illness. Symptoms of chronic, difficult cancer can be controlled by ongoing, long-term treatment to slow the spread and reduce symptoms.
3. To relieve symptoms. Palliative treatment is used to bring relief to the patient by reducing symptoms of cancer that can be neither cured nor controlled.

Currently there are four standard ways to treat cancer, used singly or in combination: surgery, radiation, drug therapy (chemotherapy or hormonal therapy), and immunotherapy.

Surgery and radiation are localized treatments, aiming directly at the tumor. Chemotherapy (drug therapy) is systemic, affecting the entire body. Hormone therapy, a form of drug therapy, is also systemic, as is immunotherapy. All these treatments have physical side effects, which give rise to emotional reactions.

Besides these methods are two others that are less common: transplants and clinical trials.

Surgery

Surgery is the most widely used treatment, and one that is effective for some kinds of cancer that have not spread widely. Usually surgery is used with other treatments to stop the spread of microscopic cells that are undetected or to target remaining cells that surgery was unable to remove.

Cancer surgery is performed for any of several different reasons:

1. To diagnose the tumor. When a tumor has been found, a bit of its tissue is removed and examined under a microscope. This proce-

dure, a biopsy, is performed to determine whether the tumor is malignant or benign. In either case, the tumor needs to be removed, for benign tumors can later turn malignant.

2. To remove cancerous tissue that has not spread widely, when nearby organs or structures, like the heart or brain, will not be damaged. The visible tumor is removed, along with a wide rim (margin) of surrounding tissue that appears to be normal but might contain cancer cells. If the tumor is solid and confined, surgery alone might cure the cancer.

3. To remove (debulk) as much of a tumor as possible when it is not possible to remove all of it.

4. To insert an implant.

5. To restore function to an organ that has been partially removed.

6. To restore the appearance or function of the body (reconstruction surgery or rehabilitation) after removal of a tumor has caused disfigurement or functional problems.

7. To control symptoms and complications caused by metastasis and provide relief when cancer has spread extensively and cannot be cured (palliative surgery); for example, to remove or bypass tumor masses that are obstructing organs or pressing on the spinal column.

8. To remove benign growths that might turn into cancer.

Side Effects

Besides causing pain, surgery, particularly to remove a tumor or bypass an obstruction, can cause permanent physical changes, such as disfigurement, loss of part of the body (e.g., a breast or a limb), loss of function (e.g., normal speech, vision), or loss of fertility. Although such surgery is sometimes mutilating, disfiguring the body may be necessary to stop a metastasis that could end in death.

New Kinds of Surgery

In recent years newer kinds of surgery have been developed that offer fewer side effects and are less invasive and less extensive. Compared to traditional open surgery, other benefits are faster recovery times, shorter hospital stays, and fewer risks of complications.

Laparoscopic surgery is performed through or more small incisions through which a small scope and special surgical instruments are inserted.

Robotic surgery, a newer approach used for certain surgical procedures, is also done through a few small incisions. Instead of holding the surgical instruments, the surgeon sits at a control panel and moves them by means of a precise robotic arm.

Radiofrequency ablation (RFA) is an outpatient procedure for patients unable to undergo surgical resection. A thin needle like probe is inserted into the tumor and the tip is heated to destroy tumor cells. Cryoablation, a similar procedure, kills cancer cells by rapid freezing and thawing.

Radiation

Like surgery, radiation is a localized treatment to rid the body of malignant cells. It is very effective for some kinds of cancer. For some inoperable tumors, it is the only treatment available. Radiation beams can be aimed directly at a tumor without destroying surrounding cells. The beams do not kill cancer cells. Rather, they destroy their DNA, rendering them incapable of dividing, so they die. Although healthy surrounding cells are damaged, the body repairs them and heals quickly.

Radiation is used for several purposes:

1. As a primary treatment to destroy certain kinds of malignancies;
2. To stop the growth of certain kinds of tumors in their early stages;
3. To reduce the risk of recurrence; and
4. To reduce symptoms.

Radiation is usually used in conjunction with chemotherapy and/or surgery. Some kinds of cancer are curable with radiation alone.

Traditional radiation therapy is administered externally. Treatments are normally given 5 days a week. During the other 2 days, the body heals any damage to the surrounding cells. Damage to the cancer cells cannot be repaired.

Since high doses of radiation are likely to cause side effects, newer techniques have been developed that target radiation more effectively to minimize those effects.

For some tumors, radiation is administered internally by means of radioactive material implanted directly in the affected area.

Another new form uses several radiation beams with varying intensity from different angles that intersect to target the tumor site. Still another technique (stereotactic radiosurgery) uses a computer to focus small beams onto a tumor. This treatment is usually done only once. For some cancers another form of radiation uses positively charged particles (protons).

Side Effects

Since radiation affects both malignant and healthy cells, some side effects are likely. Their type and severity vary, depending on the part of the body being treated, the strength of the radiation, the size of the radiation field, and other drugs that are given simultaneously. Some patients experience few or no side effects at all.

The most common side effect of any radiation treatment is fatigue, which might increase as the treatment goes on. For some patients, that is the only side effect. The skin is likely to react where the radiation is aimed, with effects such as burning, redness, hardness, blistering, itching, pain, scarring, or darkening. Some patients, however, experience no burning sensation.

There are side effects in specific areas where the radiation is directed. Radiation to the head, neck, or chest can cause a sore throat, difficulty swallowing, shortness of breath, or coughing. Directed at the mouth, it causes dryness, mouth sores, or dental problems. Radiation to the jaws can affect the salivary glands and also cause mouth sores. When treatment is administered to any of these areas, a loss of appetite is not uncommon. Radiation to the abdomen may cause diarrhea, nausea, or vomiting. Directed to the testicles or the pelvis in men, it can cause loss of sperm production and erectile dysfunction. Directed to the pelvis in women, it can cause scarring or redness in the vagina. Directed to the brain (at the scalp), it may cause decreased sexual desire, temporary hair loss, and impaired ability to concentrate. Most of these reactions are temporary and reverse themselves when the treatment has ended. However, radiation to the testes or ovaries usually results in permanent sterility.

When radioactive materials are implanted into a tumor, side effects depend on the location of the implant.

Chemotherapy

Unlike surgery and radiation, which treat only a specific part of the body, chemotherapy (chemical or drug therapy) is systemic. Since it affects the entire body, it can reach cancer cells that have spread anywhere. While its drawbacks are clear, its benefits can be extraordinary. It is often used in conjunction with surgery and radiation.

There are many different kinds of chemotherapy drugs, used singly or in combination. Some destroy malignant calls; others stop their growth by preventing them from dividing. They can be administered by injection, by pill, or intravenously. The method and the choice of drugs depend on the type and stage of the cancer.

Chemotherapy is used for any of several purposes:

1. To treat cancer known to have metastasized.
2. To treat possible unidentified cancers after the known tumor has been removed by surgery or destroyed by radiation (adjuvant chemotherapy).
3. To shrink tumors before surgery or radiation. By so doing, tumors that were formerly inoperable or untreatable can be removed or destroyed. Also, since this technique makes possible less radical surgery or less extensive radiation, it is less damaging to the patient's appearance.

Side Effects

Chemotherapy drugs can be extraordinarily beneficial in cancer treatment. At the same time, they are notorious for often causing more side effects than any other kind of cancer therapy. Because these drugs can be extremely effective in killing cancer cells that are dividing rapidly, they can also kill normal cells that are dividing rapidly, notably those in the hair follicles, bone marrow, and gastrointestinal tract. The damage done to healthy cells is temporary, but it is what causes most side effects. Those effects and their severity vary considerably depending on the specific drug, dosage, length of time between treatments, and overall health of the individual receiving treatment.

After each treatment the patient has a few weeks to recover. This means that many side effects will be most severe after treatment, and the patient can expect to feel increasingly well during the break. However, chemotherapy is likely to continue for months, and the patient might well experience increasing fatigue.

The side effects listed below and others the doctor might cite are possible, not probable, results of treatment. Not everyone experiences all of them. When they do, it is helpful that patients keep in mind that they are the symptoms of the treatment, not of the cancer, and that they are temporary. They can be expected to end when the course of treatment has ended.

Many of the side effects are the result of a lowered white blood cell count. Before each treatment, a blood test is given to determine whether the patient's count is high enough for another treatment to be tolerated.

Fatigue and weakness are the most common side effects, along with the feeling of being ill. Thinning or loss of hair, even baldness, is also common. In some cases body hair is also lost. Anemia and infections can occur. Nausea and vomiting are often experienced, as is decreased appetite and changes in the senses of taste and smell. (Some patients have such negative association with chemotherapy drugs that they become nauseous as they anticipate treatment. This is a real conditioned response, with a real physical effect, not simply an idea in their heads.)

Some chemotherapy drugs cause neuropathy (injury to the peripheral nerves), typically in the fingers and toes and possibly the entire hands and feet. The patient experiences pain, numbness, tingling, or loss of sensation in the affected areas. Symptoms gradually disappear after treatment as the nerves heal, although some drugs can cause permanent neuropathy. Some drugs can cause soreness in the mouth and throat. Some might cause diarrhea. Weight change and difficulty sleeping may be experienced, as well as change in the color of the skin and nails. Chemotherapy can produce nerve and muscle effects and kidney and bladder effects, such as pain or burning when urinating, frequent urination, inability to urinate, or bloody urine. It can induce impairment in sexual and reproductive functioning: irregular menstruation or cessation of menstruation, premature menopause, decreased sexual arousal, painful intercourse, and temporary or permanent infertility. For reasons not yet known, chemotherapy can produce intellectual changes, affecting concentration, memory, and comprehension. Clearly all these changes contribute to the patient's depression and anxiety.

To some extent, most chemotherapy drugs lower the patient's blood count for about a week following treatment. This can lead to anemia and to increased susceptibility to infections. Platelets, the clotting cells in the blood, can also be lowered, leading to increased susceptibility to bruising or bleeding. Before every treatment, a simple blood test is normally taken to ascertain that the patient's blood count is at a level safe enough for another treatment. If the test shows that the blood count or platelet level is too low, treatment will be delayed for a week or the drug dosage will be reduced.

Hormonal Therapy

Another kind of drug therapy aims at adding hormones, or blocking or manipulating hormones. This therapy is used for cancers that involve hormones for their growth: breast cancer in women and prostate cancer in men.

The most common hormones are estrogen and androgens (including testosterone). Estrogen is normally secreted primarily by the ovaries and androgen by the testes. Both are responsible for secondary sex characteristics—breasts in women and facial hair in men. Both can contribute to the growth of cancer. Hormone therapy is aimed at slowing or stopping such tumor growth. This is done by administering hormones of the opposite sex: female hormones to men and male hormones to women.

Besides breast and prostate cancer, this therapy is also used to treat uterine cancer, lymphomas, thyroid cancer, and leukemia. Hormone therapy is often used after surgery, or with radiation, chemotherapy, or both. Drugs are taken orally or by injection.

Side Effects

Men taking estrogen might experience impotence, reduced sex drive, hot flashes, or breast tenderness or growth. Long-term use can result in weight gain and bone thinning. Women taking androgens might experience sexual difficulty and discomfort and heavier hair growth. Other possible effects are weight gain, nausea, hot flashes, and fluid retention. Hormone treatment can cause premature menopause, and menopausal women might experience spotting or bleeding. It can also cause decreased sexual interest and painful intercourse. Some of these reactions can be treated, and many of them disappear when treatment is discontinued.

Immunotherapy (Biological Therapy)

Immunotherapy, which includes a wide variety of biological approaches, attempts to stimulate the body's own natural defense system, the immune system, to destroy cancer cells.

The immune system is designed to identify and destroy foreign substances in the body. However, the immune system cannot identify cancer cells because they are not significantly different from normal cells. Immunotherapy attempts to strengthen the immune system so that it can recognize cancer cells.

This therapy might utilize any of a variety of agents and strategies to accomplish this, many from the body's own cells. Such treatments include interferon or interleukin-2, which are components of the immune system, or various vaccines to stimulate immune response. Research is still ongoing as new agents and methods are being tried.

Side Effects

Weakness and fatigue are not uncommon. Patients might also feel depression. Immunotherapy can also cause difficulty thinking clearly.

Bone Marrow or Stem Cell Transplants

Transplants involve replacing defective bone marrow with healthy bone marrow. Bone marrow contains stem cells, immature blood cells that will develop into red or white cells or platelets. This treatment is used for treating some kinds of leukemia, Hodgkin's and non-Hodgkin's lymphoma, and multiple myeloma. As the result of receiving very high doses of chemotherapy, radiation, or both, the body loses the ability to make blood cells. Stem cells are part of the immune system, so that transplanting new stem cells into the bone marrow restores that ability. Transplants are accomplished either by using the patient's own stem cells or those of a donor whose tissues closely match those of the patient.

In preparation for the transplant, the patient is placed in isolation to prevent infection and subjected to very high doses of chemotherapy or high doses of total body radiation to destroy cancer cells. The procedure goes on for 6 to 8 weeks, at the end of which the marrow is injected. Because of the high doses of chemotherapy or radiation, this treatment is regarded as the most difficult of all cancer treatments for patients to undergo.

Side Effects

As a result of high-dose chemotherapy to lower the white blood cell count, the patient is at risk for various kinds of infections, bleeding, and rejection of the marrow. In rare cases, donor cells might attack the patient's immune system, causing problems with the skin, liver, or intestinal tract.

Hyperthermia

Hyperthermia is a heat treatment. Because tumor cells are more sensitive to heat than normal cells, raising the temperature is a way to try to shrink or even eradicate them. Heat, applied either externally by various means or internally, has been used for advanced breast cancer, melanoma, certain types of cervical cancer, and advanced tumors involving lymph nodes.

Hyperthermia is used along with radiation and chemotherapy in the United States, but as a stand-alone treatment abroad.

New Therapies

- Angiogenesis inhibitors are drugs designed to cut off blood supply to tumors and shrink or kill them.
- Growth-factor inhibitors are drugs to stop tumor cells from growing out of control.
- Monoclonal antibodies, produced in a laboratory rather than by the body's immune system, are drugs that attach themselves to cancer cells and attack them by preventing them from growing.
- Stereotactic radiosurgery is high-dose tightly focused radiation therapy. Using computer software and multiple beams of radiation, it damages cancer cells so they cannot reproduce, and in time they shrink. Causing minimal harm to surrounding tissues, it is often given in just one dose.
- Minimally invasive video-assisted surgery makes it possible to remove tumors with smaller incisions, less bleeding, less pain, and a shorter recovery period.

Clinical Trials

Cancer treatments used today are the result of laboratory research and clinical studies with a large number of cancer patients for long periods of time. When a drug or technique appears promising after laboratory studies, it is tested on patients. Clinical trials are research studies designed to investigate experimental cancer treatments that appear promising, but whose effectiveness and safety have not yet been demonstrated.

Clinical trials are classified into phases (1, 2, and 3), and it is important that patients and families considering a trial understand the differences between them.

Phase 1 trials are preliminary studies designed to determine how new treatments affect patients. Specifically, they are intended to assess new agents to determine the safety and any side effects that result. Since they involve the most risk, they are usually conducted only with cancer patients who have not been helped by proven treatments.

Phase 2 and 3 trials are conducted with larger numbers of patients. Phase 2 studies are intended to assess the benefits and determine dosages of the experimental treatment for different kinds of cancer. While the treatments being investigated in a phase 2 study have shown to offer some promise, it has not been established that they offer a cure. Phase 3 trials are intended to compare the experimental treatments being studied with other, already proven treatments, and to confirm their effectiveness and safety.

A clinical trial is part of the final process of research. It is through such trials that new methods are discovered and approved.

Sources

Alpha Institute. (1993). *The Alpha book on cancer and living.* Alameda, CA: Author.

American Cancer Society and CURE (2008, 2009). *Cancer resource guide.* Dallas, TX: Susan McClure.

Balch, C. (Ed.). (2008). *Cancer guide: A treatment and facilities guide for patients and their families.* Parkville, MO: Patient Resource Publishing.

Bloch, R., & Bloch, N. (1986). *Fighting cancer.* Kansas City, MO: Cancer Connection.

Buckman, R. (1997). *What you really need to know about cancer.* Baltimore, MD: Johns Hopkins University Press.

Coleman, C. N. (2006). *Understanding cancer*. Baltimore, MD: Johns Hopkins University Press.

Geffen, J. (2006). *The journey through cancer*. New York: Three Rivers Press/Crown.

Holland, J., & Lewis, S. (2001). *The human side of cancer*. New York: Quill/HarperCollins.

Ko, A., Dolinger, M., & Rosenbaum, E. (2008). *Everyone's guide to cancer therapy*. Kansas City, MO: Andrew McNeal.

Laszlo, J. (1988). *Understanding cancer*. New York: Harper and Row.

MacDonald, J. A. (1982). *When cancer strikes*. New Jersey: Prentice-Hall.

Williams, C., & Williams, S. (1986). *Cancer*. New York: Wiley Medical.

Complementary (Adjunctive) Treatments

While mainstream treatments focus on the tumor, complementary treatments are directed at enhancing the physical and mental health of the whole person. Used in conjunction with standard medical treatment, they might aim, for example, at stimulating the immune system, detoxifying the body, supplying optimum nutrition, strengthening the body, lessening the side effects of cancer treatment, lessening stress, or providing psychological help and support. They serve another purpose as well: Although patients cannot control their cancer, they can take some measure of control by choosing and seeking out complementary treatments as an adjunct to their medical program.

It was not many years ago that the medical community did not accept natural remedies and therapies as having value for healing. Now there is growing recognition of these nontraditional approaches as part of integrative treatment programs. Below is a list of the most common kinds of complementary treatments, along with brief explanations of what they are and their purposes. Further information about these and other complementary practices can be had from the National

Center for Complementary and Alternative Medicine (NCCAM), the government organization that studies these treatments, or its Web site (www.nccam.nih.gov).

Biological Protocols

These programs include the use of food, vitamin and mineral supplements, herbs, and special diets. The only kind of nutritional program recommended here is an individualized one, consisting of food and supplements, based on (1) the person's medical condition, and (2) blood tests identifying the patient's individual nutritional needs as determined by a certified nutritionist. There is no one diet or food that cures cancer, but an appropriate nutritional protocol can serve many purposes. It can strengthen the body's own healing resources during and after treatment. It can lessen the side effects of chemotherapy and radiation and improve the patient's tolerance of these treatments. It can promote more rapid recovery from surgery and increase the body's ability to resist infection. Some early research suggests that certain foods might retard the growth of cancer cells.

There are many one-size-fits-all food programs, whose use for any individual should be carefully considered. They include the macrobiotic diet, Gerson diet, and so forth. All of them have helped some people; all of them have harmed others for whom the diet was not appropriate.

Emotional and Psychological Treatments

Mainstream medicine has come to recognize that emotions and attitudes have an effect on health in both positive and negative ways. Many kinds of psychotherapy can be helpful to family members by providing emotional support and direction:

- Individual psychotherapy and counseling
- Group therapy

- Support groups
- Individual or group art therapy

Relaxation Practices

- Meditation is focused breathing or repetition of words or phrases.
- Visualization and guided imagery involve imagining experiences or visual images to relax or to facilitate healing. In visualization the person creates mental images. In guided imagery the person is directed by a facilitator or audiotape.
- Biofeedback, often used with visualization or guided imagery, is the use of a machine to aid the individual in controlling certain body functions that he is not usually aware of, such as temperature or heart rate.
- Hypnosis is an induced state of relaxation in which the person concentrates on a thought, feeling, or image.
- Yoga and tai chi are systems of gentle movement, stretches, and poses with attention given to posture, balance, concentration, and breathing.
- Aromatherapy is the use of scented plant oils to affect mood.
- Relaxation exercises are self-generated techniques, such as deep breathing, conscious muscle relaxation, and meditation to control anxiety and tension.

Physical or Body-Based Treatments

- Exercise, even in light forms such as walking, can increase energy and vitality, build strength, provide relief from stress and tension, and result in a greater sense of self-sufficiency.
- Massage, including shiatsu and Swedish massage, involves manipulation or pressure of muscles or tissues using the hands or special tools. Besides providing the emotional benefits of touch, massage can provide pain relief, improved blood flow, and heightened immune function.

- Reflexology involves massaging the acupuncture points on the feet (see acupuncture below).
- Chiropractic treatments involve manipulation of the joints or skeletal system to relieve tension and pain and promote overall vitality.
- Acupressure involves pressing one's own wrist to decrease nausea, mild discomfort, and distress.

Energy Therapies

Energy medicine rests on the belief that energy fields surround and penetrate the body and that they can be used for healing and wellness. Practitioners use pressure or move the body by putting their hands in or through these fields.

- Reiki, regarded as a spiritual rather than a physical modality, involves mentally balancing energy from a distance or placing hands on or near the body to stimulate the body's healing energy.
- Therapeutic touch involves moving hands over the body to rebalance the patient's energy.
- Qi gong involves slow movement and regulated breathing.

Bioelectromagnetics

The bioelectromagnetic approach rests on the belief that magnetic forces exist around the body. Magnets are applied to relieve chronic pain.

Medical and Healing Systems From Other Cultures

- Chinese medicine rests on the belief that health comes from a balance of two opposite forces in the body, yin and yang, and that illness is an imbalance between them. To restore balance and target the life force (qi), Chinese medicine uses various methods including herbal preparations, massage, diet, meditation, and acupuncture.

- Acupuncture, widely used in Chinese medicine, is based on the view that energy flowing through the body controls health, and that illness indicates a blockage of that flow. Acupuncture involves inserting tiny needles at specific points on the body to stimulate the natural flow of energy. It can help to promote healing, minimize pain, and, studies have shown, lessen the side effects of cancer treatment.
- Ayurvedic medicine, a system from India, views illness as imbalance. Its methods aim at restoring the natural balance between body, mind, and spirit.
- Homeopathic medicine, based on the principle that "like cures like," involves the use of small, highly diluted doses of substances that cause the body to promote healing. Those substances are similar to those which, used at higher doses, would cause the symptoms. Homeopathy may be helpful for depression, anxiety, insomnia, and side effects of cancer treatment.
- Naturopathic medicine uses natural healing forces within the body to stimulate the body to heal itself. Naturopathic practices can include diet, massage, and acupuncture.

Sources

Alpha Institute. (1993). *The Alpha book on cancer and living.* Alameda, CA: Author.

Bognar, D. (1998). *Cancer: Increasing your odds for survival.* Alameda, CA: Hunter House.

Bolletino, R. C. (1997). Cancer. In Watkins, A. (Ed.), *Mind-body medicine: A clinician's guide to psychoneuroimmunology* (pp. 87–111). Edinburgh, UK: Churchill-Livingston.

Fink, J. (1997). *Third opinion.* Toronto, Ontario: Fireside.

Geffen, J. (2006). *The journey through cancer.* New York: Random House.

Holland, J. C., & Lewis, S. (2001). *The human side of cancer.* New York: Quill/HarperCollins.

Lerner, M. (1994). *Choices in healing*. Cambridge, MA: MIT Press.

Moss, R. W. (1992). *Cancer therapy*. New York: Equinox.

Alternative Treatments

The truly alternative treatments to conventional Western medicine are the systems from other cultures listed above. There are, however, a wide variety of other alternative approaches to cancer. These treatments, usually nontoxic, are used in place of (not in addition to) conventional medical treatment. They have been validated in varying degrees by research and anecdotal evidence and have not been scientifically proven to work for large numbers of patients. For this reason they are not approved by conventional medicine. Success rates vary widely. What works for one patient may be ineffective for another. Some people for whom conventional treatments have not worked have been helped, even healed, by alternative treatments. Research studies that have investigated such therapies report a success rate of 4–10%, which included cases regarded as terminal.

It is reasonable for anyone faced with an illness that might be fatal to seek out any treatment that might conceivably help. Alternative therapies are appealing because they are "natural" and relatively nontoxic, and do not result in the discomfort and unpleasant side effects that medical treatments do. However, it is risky to substitute alternative treatments for conventional ones. Some are dangerous, many are expensive, and, if they don't work, patients who try them can lose precious time during which they could have been benefiting from conventional treatments. Anyone considering an alternative treatment should obtain all possible information about it.

Only patients can decide what is best for them. The treatment chosen should be the one offering the best odds of getting better, not the one that is the most gentle. There are various kinds of alternative approaches, including the three described below.

- Dietary therapies include the macrobiotic diet, which is largely vegetarian and low on calories and protein; the Gerson regimen, consisting of a largely vegetarian diet, various pharmaceutical agents, and the use of coffee enemas; and wheatgrass therapy, combining the use of wheatgrass juice with a diet of raw fruits and vegetables, sprouted grains, nuts and seeds, and greens.
- Herbal treatments.
- Pharmacological and biological approaches, a diverse group of alternative treatments that have as their central component substances such as biochemical agents, vaccines, blood products, and synthetic chemicals.

Sources

Fink, J. (1997). *Third opinion*. Toronto, Ontario: Fireside.

Lerner, M. (1996). *Choices in healing*. Cambridge, MA: MIT Press.

Morra, M., & Potts, E. (1987). *Choices: Realistic alternatives in cancer treatment*. Dresden, TN: Avon.

Moss, R. W. (1992). *Cancer therapy*. New York: Equinox.

Pelton, R., & Overholser, L. (1994). *Alternatives in cancer therapy*. New York: Simon & Schuster.

Psychological Side Effects of Treatments

Being told that you have a life-threatening illness is itself an emotional trauma. With physical pain, the trauma is more severe. Added to the illness itself, the experience of receiving surgery, radiation, or chemotherapy—as well as the physical side effects of such treatments—predictably cause strong emotional reactions. Some cancer treatments have psychological as well as physical side effects.

People most at risk for severe psychological symptoms are:

- Those who are having or had prolonged treatment or extensive hospital stays (such as patients receiving bone marrow transplants).
- Those being treated for a cancer recurrence.
- Those with previous emotional trauma, particularly a history that includes victimization.
- Those with previous psychological problems.
- Those with a family member who died of cancer.
- Those grieving the recent death of someone close.
- Those who, at the time of diagnosis, were experiencing some kind of major loss or setback in their life.

In some individuals, cancer might ignite old symptoms of posttraumatic stress or cause new ones, replete with nightmares and flashbacks at any time before, during, or after treatment. Pain itself from the illness or the treatment can produce such psychological effects as irritability, anxiety, sadness, depression, and insomnia.

Cancer treatment is physically and psychologically difficult for anyone. When the going gets rough, patients might well become ambivalent. They know that treatment is necessary but at the same time, when they feel sick or in pain, they might feel resistant to continuing with it. For this reason alone, it is important that they are given time to make treatment decisions. The ideal here is that they fully understand their options, discuss them with their physicians and families, and make decisions so that they can be confident about the protocol chosen. What is wanted is that they can commit to it, not submit. If they lack confidence, their experience in treatment, as well as their adjustment and recovery, will be far more difficult.

Surgery

When surgery is planned, most patients and their families experience anticipatory fear, anxiety, and even dread, along with such associated physical symptoms as dry mouth and shortness of breath. Patients fear being cut open, being put to sleep, and possibly not waking up. They fear being in pain.

Psychological reactions before and after the surgery are far more intense if the surgery is certain to have a major impact on the person's life by resulting in the loss of a body part or of normal functioning. Such traumatizing operations include those involving the removal of a limb, a breast, or the voice box; those affecting sexual or reproductive functioning; and those involving removal of the bladder, colon, or intestine along with the creation of an opening in the abdominal wall requiring the use of a bag for elimination. Any such surgery that disfigures the body, such as mastectomy or colostomy, is an attack on the person's identity, and can affect their way of life and their relationships. Feeling unattractive, unlovable, and sexually undesirable, patients might experience decreased sexual desire, as well as depression and even despair.

Chemotherapy

The first psychological effects—anxiety, fear, and dread—often are experienced long before the first treatment begins, as soon as it has been decided that the patient will receive chemotherapy. Patients and families are anxious about what the treatment will be, what side effects will be experienced, and how they can cope as the patient becomes weaker and sick.

It is helpful for them to be aware that physical side effects vary considerably, depending on the drug or drug combination received. Some drugs almost invariably produce strong physical side effects; some cause only relatively minimal reactions. Another factor is the treatment schedule. Since chemotherapy is usually administered in a 3- or 4-week cycle, side effects gradually lessen after each treatment as the patient recovers. It is also helpful for them to be aware that many side effects can be minimized—for example, with medications—and that when the treatment has ended, normally all physical side effects gradually disappear.

For the most part, psychological reactions to chemotherapy drugs occur in direct proportion to the severity of physical side effects. Feeling frequent fatigue, nausea, neuropathy, weakness, or flulike symptoms is clearly depressing. Further, chemotherapy agents affect the ability to think clearly and to concentrate. This physical effect can cause emotional reactions. Fear, anxiety, irritability, depression, and mood swings are common. Patients complain of having no control of their emotions, finding themselves at times bursting into tears or lashing out in irritation. Besides the fatigue caused by chemotherapy drugs, the patient might experience insomnia, resulting in further fatigue, which can exacerbate such emotional reactions.

Repeated treatments can result in anticipatory nausea, even vomiting, shortly before subsequent treatments. That is, the patient might feel sick when entering the treatment center or sooner, simply in anticipation of the next treatment. This reaction is not simply in the patient's head. It is a conditioned response, with physical manifestations.

Other Drug Treatments

Some drugs, notably steroids or pain medications, can produce dramatic changes in mood, intellectual functioning, and behavior. Drugs that disturb hormone balance (hormone treatment) can affect sexual desire.

Radiation

As with almost all cancer treatments, many patients feel fearful and apprehensive before treatments begin. They fear radiation and the effects they expect it to have on them. The treatments themselves, however, usually cause minimal changes in mood and emotion. Emotional reactions that do occur, such as sadness and depression, generally appear to result not from the treatment itself but from the fact of having cancer and undergoing radiation treatments daily.

Other psychological reactions can occur in response to physical effects of the treatment. Notably, radiation to the brain can impair concentration and short-term memory.

Bone Marrow Transplants

Because of the high doses of chemotherapy drugs or radiation required, bone marrow transplants are the most rigorous cancer treatment available and, for the patient, the most arduous, stressful, and difficult, physically and emotionally. For a patient to undergo the weeks of treatment before the marrow is administered, great emotional stamina and determination are required. While the procedure also entails high risks, it is usually effective. It is used when no other treatment is likely to offer the same long-term benefits.

Immunotherapy

Patients often feel depression, sometimes extreme depression, which is apparently the effect of immunotherapy drugs on the brain as well as the response to extreme weakness and fatigue. When these drugs are administered in high doses, patients also have difficulty thinking clearly.

Sources

Holland, J. C., & Lewis, S. (2001). *The human side of cancer*. New York: Quill/HarperCollins.

Seligman, L. (1996). *Promoting a fighting spirit*. San Francisco: Jossey-Bass.

Some Techniques for Managing Stress

Meditation

Meditating can promote physical and emotional relaxation and calmness. By providing practice in focusing on the present moment, it can serve as a useful technique for letting go of fears, anxiety, and concerns. The state of calm induced by meditation can also lead to clarity of thought and new insights. Meditation involves concentrating on something external (repeating a word or phrase aloud or focusing on an object) or something internal (silently reciting a prayer or a repeated word, phrase, or question; or imagining a memory or a visual image). The objective is to concentrate only on the chosen focus of attention and nothing else while remaining awake and alert.

Meditation is most helpful when it is practiced regularly, once or twice a day, for 10, 15, or 20 minutes, ideally at the same time of day and in the same place. It can also be used in stress situations (for example, in the dentist's chair) to promote relaxation.

To begin any meditation or visualization, sit or lie in a comfortable position. Close your eyes. Breathe naturally and allow your muscles to relax. With every breath, let go of more and more tension.

Meditation 1: Breath Counting

As you breathe, count your exhalations until you get to four. When you reach four, go back to one, and continue to count. You can focus on the sound of your breathing or the physical feeling of breathing, or you can visualize the numbers. Use whatever mode is the natural one for you.

Whenever anything comes into your mind other than your breathing—a thought, a sound you hear, a physical sensation, a feeling—let it go and bring yourself gently back to the counting.

Whenever you are distracted (and you can be sure that you will be), bring yourself back to the counting. Whatever thoughts you have, just let them come and go, without judging them or judging yourself for having them. (No matter how long you practice meditation, you will continue to be distracted again and again.)

When you bring yourself back, do so gently, lovingly, and compassionately, with the understanding that you didn't fail at meditating. You were distracted only because that is the nature of the human mind.

Meditation 2: Repetition of Your Own Special Word or Phrase

Choose any word or phrase that has a special and positive meaning for you. The word can be in any language, from any religious or spiritual tradition. If you prefer, instead of a word choose any soothing sound that you find to be pleasant.

Concentrate on your chosen word or phrase, then repeat it again and again aloud or silently. You might want to coordinate the words with your breathing.

Whenever you find yourself drifting from your special words, distracted by a sound, a thought, a feeling, or a sensation, bring yourself back gently and continue with the meditation until the end of the allotted time.

A Visualization

Imagine yourself doing something active that you enjoy. You might visualize yourself running along a beach, swimming, walking through a forest, skiing, or whatever comes to mind that you would like to do and where you would like to do it.

Now try to imagine how you would feel doing it. Imagine the carefree feeling of freedom, strength, and energy you have.

Intensify that image to make it as vivid as possible. Imagine how your body feels as you move. Imagine the feeling of the sun or the wind on your face. See the beautiful, natural colors of the earth, the sky, the trees, or the water, and try to hear all the sounds.

Stay with that visualization as long as you like.

When you are ready to come back, imagine locking that image into your mind and heart, so it is there for your mind and your body to direct your energies toward.

A Meditative Visualization: Safe Harbor

This is a self-guided visualization. Very often in stressful times we tell ourselves that life has always been difficult—but in fact this is not true. For all of us there have been wonderful moments. This visualization is to remind you of those times and of how you felt when they happened.

It can be helpful to precede this with 5 or 10 minutes of breath counting.

Imagine that you are in a gray place—that is, don't try to visualize anything.

Now invite your mind or consciousness to send up a memory of a time, from any period of your life, when you felt safe and secure, when you felt completely like yourself, when you didn't want to change a thing. It might be a time when you were alone or with someone else. (If such a memory does not come up right away, just wait.)

When you have that memory, try to re-create it, intensifying it, to make it as vivid as possible. For example, if your memory is of walking on an ocean beach, how did the air feel? What sounds did you hear? Try to imagine the sounds of the gulls and the waves. What did you feel? How did the sand feel under your feet? How did the sun feel on your body?

Relive that memory as fully as you can. Spend as much time in that memory as you like, and when you are finished with it, let it go.

Go back into the gray place, invite another such memory, and wait.

Do this again, with as many or as few memories as you like, until your meditation time is over.

Before opening your eyes, imagine that you are taking the feelings you had during the times you just imagined and locking them inside you so that the feelings the memories bring are always there for you to recall easily.

A Visualization for Relaxation

Imagine that with every exhalation you are breathing out any tension you are holding. Let the various parts of your body relax more and more. Feel them relax fully and completely.

Allow yourself to drift off into a place you imagine—your own special place where you are safe and relaxed. Your place might be an ocean beach, a meadow, a mountain lake, a quiet forest, a garden, or anywhere you feel safe and relaxed.

Notice how the sun is warming your body and a gentle breeze touches you lightly, as warm relaxation flows over you. Your face is relaxing, your neck, arms, shoulders, chest, stomach, hips, back, and legs. All you have to do is lie there and let the relaxation flow over you.

Whenever you feel ready, open your eyes and feel rested, more alert than before.

Concentrated Muscle Relaxation

Notice if you are holding tension anywhere in your body, if you are gritting your teeth, for example, or whether your shoulders are tense.

Take a deep breath and relax.

Grip something close to you—the arms of a chair, for example—and squeeze as hard as you can.

Imagine that all the tension in your body is moving to your hands.

Continue to grip hard for a few moments.

Let go and relax. As you let go, imagine that all the tension is floating out of your body and away, like a balloon floating into the sky.

Progressive Muscle Relaxation

This is a systematic procedure of tensing and relaxing all your muscles in a given sequence. This practice, used to relieve anxiety, can be done sitting up or lying down. By practicing tensing muscles and then relaxing them, you learn to become aware of any tension you are holding in some part your body, as well as the feeling of relaxation.

Bend your arms and hold your fists up in front of you at about shoulder level. Now clench your fists in a tight ball. Hold, hold, hold, and then let go. Let your arms drop at your sides or into your lap. Relax.

Now close your eyes and screw up the muscles in your face, including your forehead. Hold that tension for about 5 seconds. Then let it go. Relax.

Open your mouth wide, as wide as you can, and hold it open in a big yawn. Hold for three counts and then relax.

Tense your neck muscles. Hold for about 5 seconds, then relax.

Drop your chin down to your chest. Move your head around so that your ear touches or almost touches your right shoulder. Bring your head around to the back, down to your left shoulder, down to the front again, and then up.

Repeat, moving in the opposite direction: move your chin from your chest to your left shoulder, tilt back, around to your right shoulder, and down to the front again. Relax.

Shrug both shoulders, bringing them up toward your ears as high as you can. Hold them there, hold, then let them drop and relax.

Clasp your hands and stretch your arms out straight in front of you tightly. Hold them there for a few seconds, then let go and relax.

Clasp your hands and stretch your arms straight out behind you. Hold for a few seconds, then relax and let them go.

Tighten the muscles in your abdomen and buttocks. Hold, then relax.

Tighten the muscles in your thighs and calves. Hold, then relax.

Stretch your legs straight out in front of you, with toes pointed outward. Hold, then relax.

Stretch your legs straight out in front of you, with toes pointed inward. Hold, then relax.

Complementary Treatments That Can Ease Pain and Discomfort

P*hysical Manipulation*, such as massage or movement of painful areas, can help muscle pain.

Movement Therapies, such as yoga, physical therapy, and Tai Chi, can help with pain in the muscles, lower back, and joints.

Energy Healing, such as acupuncture, acupressure, Qi Gong and Reiki, can help with pain caused by injuries or complicated by anxiety, depression, or trauma.

Nutritional Programs and Herbal Remedies can increase the body's immunity, reduce pain caused by inflammation, and help with insomnia. A nutritional program might include, for example, anti-inflammatory diets high in fresh fruit, vegetables, whole grains, fish, and olive oil. Supplements might include Omega-3-fatty acids to reduce inflammation. Herbal remedies might include ginger root to inhibit pain, or turmeric to reduce inflammation.

Meditation, Imagery, and Relaxation can sometimes ease many kinds of chronic pain.

Lifestyle Changes, such as exercise, changes in work or relationships, or more time spent in enjoyable activities, can help with many kinds of chronic pain.

Sources

Alpha Institute. (1998). *The Alpha book on cancer and living*. Alameda, CA: Author.

AARP Magazine Health Report. January–February 2009: 26–30.

Bognar, D. (1998). *Cancer: Increasing your odds for survival*. Alameda, CA: Hunter House.

Bolletino, R. C. (1997). "Cancer." In Watkins, A. (Ed.). *Mind-Body Medicine: A Clinician's Guide to Psychoneuroimmunology*. New York, NY: Churchill Livingstone.

Some Legal and Practical Preparations When the Patient Is Dying

Advance Directives

A person who is seriously ill may well become incapacitated and no longer able to make medical and financial decisions. Preparing for that eventuality is important for the patient's and family's peace of mind.

Living Will

Medical science has the technology to keep people alive for an indefinite time. Most people do not want to linger in a long dying process with no hope of recovery. They would choose to die rather than to be sustained by machines. In some hospitals, artificial life support is given automatically to prolong life if the patients have not prepared a written document expressing their decision against it. A living will, prepared by a competent patient, communicates to physicians the patient's wishes about life-support equipment and other extraordinary measures that can prolong life.

There is an extremely important reason to arrange for such a directive. In some states in the United States, prolonging life in patients with no hope of recovery is the only legally sanctioned course of treatment. Treatment can be withdrawn or withheld only according to a living will signed by the patient, or "clear and convincing evidence" of the patient's wishes. Some states, to varying extents, allow relatives, friends, or guardians to make decisions about life support.

Decisions about advance directives are not always easy to reach and are best made through discussions and agreements with the patient, the family, and physicians. The medical team needs to know the patient and family's wishes about treatment decisions.

A living will prepared by the patient absolves family members of the burden of making decisions without knowing what the patient wanted and also absolves physicians of the burden of having to decide whether to administer artificial life support. A Do Not Resuscitate order can be put in place by doctors, but only if there are no identified surrogates, and only if resuscitation is considered futile.

Durable Power of Attorney for Health Care (Health Care Proxy)

Not all doctors or hospitals recognize living wills, and sometimes the legality of these directives is challenged. For that reason, the patient might want to appoint a legal health care proxy, a trusted person who will make decisions about treatment and medical care should the patient be unable to do so.

Power of Attorney

A number of circumstances can arise that make it highly advisable for a family member or someone the patient trusts to have power of attorney, which is the legal right to make decisions or sign for the patient when the patient is unable to do so. The patient might be highly medicated or in a coma when medical tests or surgery are needed, and decisions might have to be made quickly. The patient might be unable to sign a bank or insurance check when the family needs to deposit the funds.

Will

A will states the patient's wishes for the settlement of his estate. It specifies the distribution of personal belongings and assets, and provides for family needs, including, if necessary, naming a guardian for minor children.

Without a will, the state can determine how an estate is settled. Its determination can leave a spouse or children with only a small portion of the patient's assets. Requirements vary from one state to another. To ensure that these documents are valid, they should be drawn up by an attorney.

References

Alpha Institute. (1998). *The Alpha book on cancer and living*. Alameda, CA: Author.

American Cancer Society and CURE. (2008, 2009). *Cancer resource guide*. Dallas, TX: Cure Media Group.

American Psychiatric Association. (1994). *Diagnostic and statistical manual of mental disorders* (4th ed.). Washington, DC: Author.

Anderson, G. (1999) *Cancer: 50 essential things to do*. New York: Plume.

Ascher, B. L. (1993). *Landscape without gravity*. New York: Penguin.

Babcock, E. D. (1997). *When life becomes precious*. New York: Bantam.

Balch, C. M. (Ed.). (2008, Spring/Summer). *Patient resource cancer guide*. Parkville, MO: Patient Resource Publishing.

Benjamin, H. H. (1987). *From victim to victor*. New York: Dell.

Blake, W. (1992). *Songs of innocence and songs of experience*. Mineola, NY: Dover.

Bolletino, R. C. (1996). Response to "Can the self affect the course of cancer?" *Advances: The Journal of Mind-Body Health, 12*(4), 72–74.

Bolletino, R. C. (1997). Cancer. In A. Watkins (Ed.), *Mind-body medicine: A clinician's guide to psychoneuroimmunology* (pp. 87–111). Edinburgh, UK: Churchill-Livingston.

Bolletino, R. C. (1998). The need for a new ethical model in medicine:

A challenge for conventional, alternative and complementary practitioners. *Advances in Mind-Body Medicine, 14*(1), 16–28.

Bolletino, R. C. (2001). A model of spirituality for psychotherapy and other fields of mind-body medicine. *Advances in Mind-Body Medicine, 17*(2), 90–107.

Bolletino, R. C. (2004). The patient as a person and research studies. *Integrative Cancer Therapies, 3*(20), 163–179.

Boss, J. (2000). *Ambiguous loss.* Cambridge, MA: Harvard University Press.

Bowers, M. K., Jackson, E. N., Knight, J. A., & LeShan, L. (1964). *Counseling the dying.* New York: Thomas Nelson.

Brody, J. (2008, August 19). Cancer therapy: There is a time to treat and a time to let go. *New York Times.*

Brown, T. (2008, September 9). If death is proud, more reason to savor life. *New York Times,* F1.

Broyard, A. (1992). *Intoxicated by my illness.* New York: Fawcett Columbine.

Buber, M. (1990). *Hasidism and modern man.* M. S. Jaffee (Ed.). Philadelphia: University of Pennsylvania Press.

Caine, L. (1990). *Being a widow.* New York: Penguin.

Campbell, J. (1991). *Reflections on the art of living: A Joseph Campbell companion* (D. K. Osbon, Ed.). New York: Harper Collins.

Carroll, L. (1991). *Through the looking glass* (D. J. Grey, Ed.). New York: W.W. Norton.

Cassell, E. J. (1994). *The nature of suffering and the goals of medicine.* New York: Oxford University Press.

Coles, R. (2002). A young psychiatrist looks at his profession. In R. Coles & R. Testa (Eds.), *A life in medicine.* New York: New Press.

Conrad, J. (1988). *Lord Jim.* New York: Penguin Classics.

Cousins, N. (1986). New foreword. In D. T. Jafee, *Healing from within.* New York: Simon and Schuster.

Cousins, N. (1989). *Head first: The biology of hope.* New York: E. P. Dutton.

Cousins, N. (1990). Foreword. In N. A. Fiore, *The road back to health.* Berkeley, CA: Celestial Arts.

Cunningham, A. J. (2005). *Can the mind heal cancer? A clinician-scientist examines the evidence.* Toronto, Canada: Alastair J. Cunningham.

Daudet, A. (2002). *In the land of pain* (J. Barnes, Trans.). London: Jonathan Cape.

Devries, M. (1993). *Choosing life: A new perspective on illness and healing.* Helen Dowling Institute for Biopsychosocial Medicine. Lisse, Netherlands: Swets & Zeitlinger.

Doherty, W. (1999a). Morality and spirituality in therapy. In F. Walsh (Ed.), *Spiritual resources in family therapy.* New York: Guilford.

Doherty, W. (1999b). *Soul searching: Why psychotherapy must promote moral responsibility.* New York: Basic Books.

Dossey, L. (1992). *Meaning and medicine.* San Francisco: Harper San Francisco.

Duff, K. (1992). *The alchemy of illness.* New York: Penguin.

Einstein, A. (1982). *Ideas and opinions* (S. Bargmann, Trans.). New York: Crown.

Eliot, T. S. (1952). The love song of J. Alfred Prufrock. In *T. S. Eliot: The complete poems and plays.* New York: Harcourt, Brace.

Eliot, T. S. (1964). *The elder statesman.* New York: Noonday Press.

Emerson, R. W. (1860). *The conduct of life essays.* New York: Doubleday.

Fiore, N. A. (1990). *The road back to health.* Berkeley, CA: Celestial Arts.

Fitzgerald, F. S. (1964). *The crack-up.* New York: W.W. Norton.

Fitzgerald, H. (1999). *The grieving child.* New York: Simon and Schuster.

Ford, J. (1968). *The broken heart.* Lincoln, NE: University of Nebraska Press.

Frank, J. D. (1991). *Persuasion & healing.* Baltimore, MD: Johns Hopkins University Press.

Frankl, V. (1959). *From death camp to existentialism*. Boston: Beacon.

Frankl, V. (1983). *The doctor and the soul*. New York: Vintage Books.

Frankl, V. (1985). *The unheard cry for meaning*. New York: Washington Square Press.

Frankl, V. (1992). *Man's search for meaning*. Boston: Beacon.

Frankl, V. (1995). *Psychotherapy and existentialism*. New York: Washington Square Press.

Fromm-Reichmann, F. (1960). *Principles of intensive therapy*. Chicago: University of Chicago Press.

Gide, A. (1987). *The journals of Andre Gide, Vol. 2: 1924-1949*. (J. O'Brien, Ed. & Trans). Evanston, IL: Northwestern University Press. (Original work published 1892)

Girard, V. (2001). *There's no place like hope*. Lynnwood, WA: Vickie Girard and Compendium.

Glaser, W. (1975). *Reality therapy: A new approach to psychiatry*. New York: Harper & Row.

Goldie, L. (2005). *Psychotherapy and the treatment of cancer patients*. New York: Routledge.

Groopman, J. (2003). *The anatomy of hope*. New York: Random House.

Heiney, S. P., Hermann, J. F., Bruss, K. V., & Fincannon, J. L. (2005). *Cancer in the family: Helping children cope with a parent's illness*. Atlanta, GA: American Cancer Society.

Herman, J. L. (1992). *Trauma and recovery*. New York: Basic Books.

Hillel. (1975). *Ethics of the Talmud, sayings of the fathers*. New York: Schocken Press.

Holland, J. C., & Lewis, S. (2001). *The human side of cancer*. New York: Quill/HarperCollins.

Holt, J. (2007, January 21). You are what you expect. *New York Times Magazine*, 15-16.

Hope, L. (2005). *Help me live: 20 things people with cancer want you to know*. Berkeley, CA: Celestial Arts.

Housman, A. E. (1940). *Last poems*. New York: Henry Holt.

Hudson, C. (1990). Authenticity and flexibility. In D. Roth & E. Levier (Eds.), *Being human in the face of death*. Santa Monica, CA: IBS Press.

Jackson, E. (1983). *Coping with the crisis in your life*. Northvale, NJ: Jason Aronson.

Jourard, S. (1964). *The transparent self*. Princeton, NJ: Van Nostrand.

Jourard, S. (1968). *Disclosing man to himself*. Princeton, NJ: Van Nostrand.

Jourard, S. (1971). *The transparent self* (2nd ed.). Princeton, NJ: Van Nostrand.

Jung, C. G. (1965). *Memories, dreams and reflections* (A. Jaffe, Ed.). New York: Vintage Books.

Jung, C. G. (1978). *Psychological reflections* (J. Jacobi and R. F. C. Hull, Eds.). Princeton, NJ: Princeton University Press.

Jung, C. G. (1989). Psychotherapy Today. In *Essays on contemporary events* (R. F. C. Hull, Trans.). Princeton, NJ: Princeton University Press.

Kane, J. (2003). *How to heal: A guide for caregivers*. New York: Helios Press.

Klopfer, B. (1951). Psychological variables in human cancer. *Journal of Projective Techniques, 12*(4), 331–340.

Kübler-Ross, E. (1969). *On death and dying*. New York: Macmillan.

Kübler-Ross, E. (1987). *Working it through*. New York: Macmillan.

Kübler-Ross, E. (1989). The four pillars of healing. In R. Carlson & B. Shield (Eds.), *Healers on healing*. Los Angeles: Jeremy Tarcher.

Kübler-Ross, E., & Kessler, D. (2005). *On grief and grieving*. New York: Scribner.

Laing, R. D. (1982). *The voice of experience*. New York: Parthenon.

Lerner, M. (1996). *Choices in healing*. Cambridge, MA: MIT Press.

LeShan, E. (1996). *When a parent is very sick*. Boston: Atlantic Monthly Press.

LeShan, L. (1964). The patient in severe pain of long duration. *Journal of Chronic Diseases, 17*, 119–120.

LeShan, L. (1980). *You can fight for your life*. New York: M. Evans.

LeShan, L. (1982). *The mechanic and the gardener.* New York: Holt, Rinehart and Winston.

LeShan, L. (1992). Creating a climate for self-healing: The principles of modern psychosomatic medicine. *Advances, 8*(4), 20–27.

LeShan, L. (1994). *Cancer as a turning point.* New York: Plume.

LeShan, L. (1996). *Beyond technique.* Northvale, NJ: Jason Aronson.

LeVert, S. (1995). *When someone you love has cancer.* New York: Dell.

Lewis, C. S. (1975). *A grief observed.* New York: Bantam.

Lochner, C. (1990a). Journeying side by side. In D. Roth & E. Levier (Eds.), *Being human in the face of death.* Santa Monica, CA: IBS Press.

Lochner, C. (1990b). Being fully present. In D. Roth & E. Levier (Eds.), *Being human in the face of death.* Santa Monica, CA: IBS Press.

Lorde, A. (1980). *The cancer journals.* San Francisco: Aunt Lute Books.

Luther, M. (1993). *Psalms with introduction by Martin Luther.* St. Louis, MO: Concordia.

MacDonald, J. A. (1982). *When cancer strikes.* Englewood Cliffs, NJ: Prentice Hall.

Mann, T. (1981). *The Magic Mountain.* (H. T. Lowe-Porter, Trans.). Franklin, PA: Franklin Library.

Matte, G. (2001). *When the body says no: Understanding the stress-disease connection.* Hoboken, NJ: John Wiley.

Milne, A. A. (1997). *The complete tales and poems of Winnie-the-Pooh.* New York: Dutton.

Moore, T. E. (1998). Spiritualities of depth. *Tikkun,* (November–December).

Needleman, J. (1977). *The new religions.* New York: Dutton.

Nordenberg, T. The healing power of placebos. *FDA Consumer Magazine, 34*(1).

Pomeroy, D. (1996). *When someone you love has cancer.* New York: Berkeley Books.

Prather, J. (1989). What Is Healing? In R. Carlson and B. Shield (Eds.), *Healers on healing.* Los Angeles: Jeremy Tarcher.

Proust, M. (1970). *Remembrance of things past, Vol. 6: The sweet cheat gone*. New York: Random House.

Roethke, T. (1948). The lost son, "It was beginning winter." In *The lost son and other poems*. Garden City, NY: Doubleday.

Rosak, T. (1995). *The making of a counter-culture*. Berkeley, CA: University of California. (Original work published 1969)

Rouseau, J.-J. (1964). *Emile, Julie and other writings*. Woodbury, NY: Barron's Educational Series.

Schweitzer, A. (1998). *Out of my life and thought* (A. J. Lemke, Trans.). Baltimore: Johns Hopkins University Press.

Seligman, L. (1996). *Promoting a fighting spirit*. San Francisco, CA: Jossey-Bass.

Siegel, B. (1998). *Love, medicine & miracles*. New York: Harper Perennial.

Simonton, S. M. (1989). *The healing family*. New York: Bantam Books.

Sontag, S. (1990). *Illness as metaphor and AIDS and its metaphor*. New York: Anchor Books/Doubleday.

Sweeney, T. J. (2000). Learning to be a caregiver, trying to be a brother. In C. Levine (Ed.), *Always on call*. New York: United Hospital Fund of New York.

Swinburne, A. C. (1936). The garden of proserpine. In M. Van Doren (Ed.), *An anthology of world poetry*. New York: Harcourt Brace.

Tolstoy, L. (1981). *The death of Ivan Ilyich* (L. Solotaroff, Trans.). New York: Bantam Books.

Ungersma, A. J. (1961). *The search for meaning: A new approach in psychotherapy and pastoral psychology*. Philadelphia: Westminster Press.

Watters, E., & Ofshe, R. (1999). *Therapy's delusions*. New York: Scribner.

Wolpe, G. I. (2000). A crisis of caregiving, a crisis of faith. In C. Levine (Ed.), *Always on call*. New York: United Hospital Fund of New York.

Wordsworth, W. (2002). We are seven. In *Selected Poetry of William Wordsworth*. Mineola, NY: Dover.

Yalom, I. (1998). Foreword. In R. Rabinowitz (Ed.), *Inside therapy*. New York: St. Martin's Press.

Yalom, I. (2003). *The gift of therapy*. New York: HarperCollins Perennial.

Yeats, W. B. (1966). He wishes for the cloths of heaven. In *The wind among the reeds: The collected poems of W. B. Yeats*. New York: Macmillan.

Zuckerman, C. (2000). Til death do us part. In C. Levine (Ed.), *Always on call*. New York: United Hospital Fund of New York.

Index